PEARSON EDUCATION

NURSING&HEALTH

FIRST FOR HEALTH

We work with leading authors to develop the strongest
educational materials in nursing and healthcare, bringing
cutting-edge thinking and best learning practice to a
global market.

Under a range of well-known imprints, including Pearson,
we craft high-quality print and electronic publications which
help readers to understand and apply their content,
whether studying or at work.

To find out more about the complete range of our
publishing, please visit us on the World Wide Web at:
www.pearsoned.co.uk.

Introducing Psychology for Nurses and Healthcare Professionals

Professor Dominic Upton

Head of Psychological Sciences
University of Worcester

Harlow, England • London • New York • Boston • San Francisco • Toronto
Sydney • Tokyo • Singapore • Hong Kong • Seoul • Taipei • New Delhi
Cape Town • Madrid • Mexico City • Amsterdam • Munich • Paris • Milan

Pearson Education Limited
Edinburgh Gate
Harlow
Essex CM20 2JE
England

and Associated Companies throughout the world

Visit us on the World Wide Web at:
www.pearsoned.co.uk

First published 2010

© Pearson Education Limited 2010

ISBN 978-0-273-72144-4

British Library Cataloguing-in-Publication Data
A catalogue record for this book is available from the British Library

Library of Congress Cataloging-in-Publication Data

10 9 8 7 6 5 4 3 2 1
12 11 10

Typeset in 9.5/13 pt Interstate-Light by 73
Printed in Great Britain by Henry Ling Ltd., at the Dorset Press, Dorchester, Dorset

The publisher's policy is to use paper manufactured from sustainable forests.

Contents

Preface

The role of psychology in nursing education and practice has become ever more significant in recent years and some (and I am one of them) would argue that it is the most important topic you will cover during your studies. Although psychology has always had a role in the nursing curriculum (although sometimes not called psychology), in recent years this has come ever more to the fore. Even though psychology is a mandatory component of your programme, I hope that this text and the suggested additional reading will give you both an insight into, and a thirst for, psychology. More importantly, however, I hope that you will be able to use the material and the knowledge developed from this text within your practice for your clients' and patients' benefit.

The increase in interest and acknowledgement of the value of psychology has led to an increase in the number of texts, research and policy publications linking nursing, healthcare and psychology. This substantial body of literature has formed the backdrop of this book. Many (or perhaps in reality, *some*) of these publications have been read from the classic texts of yesteryear (i.e. anything before 2000!) to those more recent, including some that are not even published yet. When presenting this material, however, this text has taken an academically robust approach but attempted to do this is an appealing and readable manner. Hence, for example, even though the studies and reports have been read and reported here, the reference list has been kept to a minimum, although I hope the academic rigour that went into the preparation of this text comes through. There is a list of further reading for each of the topics and this will guide you into the deeper recesses of psychology (and I am sure you will want to go there . . .). In short, this is a text book that is academic in tone and presentation and also useful and relevant for student nurses from all backgrounds with a range of professional aspirations. In this way this text is inclusive in nature and demonstrates the importance of psychology in both the nursing role and in healthcare in general. I am passionate about psychology and, importantly, communicating its relevance and effectiveness in nursing practice. I hope that this comes through.

The aim of the text was, therefore, to be inclusive, to demonstrate the value of psychology in nursing and healthcare from a British perspective. Although there are a number of American texts dealing with psychology there are few that have a British focus. There are, of course, other texts exploring health psychology or psychology in general but these do not explicitly link psychological aspects of health to the nursing role. Therefore, we have tried in this book to cover psychological aspects and concepts that have a direct role in health and nursing care. However, this text does not claim to be comprehensive – it does not cover every single aspect of psychology, for this would be impossible; it does not even cover every single aspect of psychology related to healthcare, as this too would be impossible.

However, what has been achieved is a text that highlights the key areas in psychology related to nursing care. Every chapter has been honed to ensure that every single element is related to either your studies or your practice.

The choice, of course, is a subjective one and the decisions of what to include and what to exclude will (no doubt) be contentious – there are so many competing perspectives in psychology and its scope is so extensive (see Chapter 2 for further details). More could have been included on social groups and the nature of groupthink and social loafing (which would have helped you when working in a team) or coping with chronic illness could have been further explored or why people go to their healthcare practitioner, or the role of nurses in promoting and extending health behaviours, and many more topics besides. However, something had to give – and these (amongst other things) were them.

This book has been produced with a number of aims in mind. Firstly, for the student nurse to become familiar with how the role of psychology and health psychology can be applied to nursing and healthcare practice. Secondly, for the student nurse to be able to apply theories and ideas to both their own placement practice and student nurse portfolios. Thirdly, to do this in a simplistic but robust manner with an interactive and supportive style. Finally, to ensure that there is a commitment to the role of psychology in nursing care.

Psychology has many perspectives which enable the nurse student to appreciate the individuality and diversity of patients. This is important in the construction and delivery of individualised care plans as stated throughout nursing courses and, of course, the Nursing and Midwifery Code of Conduct. Material presented in this text includes specific material dedicated to explaining how this can be successfully achieved in practice.

Creating a patient led NHS – delivering the NHS Improvement Plan (DoH, 2005a) is a government health paper which highlights the importance of patient-centredness including patient choice and needs that should be addressed within any interaction with a patient. Hopefully, this book builds on the vision of such government statements and encourages the reader to appreciate the input psychology can have with such emerging visions of the future. There are, of course, many other policy developments that highlight the importance of a patient-centred NHS, ill-health prevention and promoting health and well-being (e.g. *Our Health, Our Care, Our Say: A New Direction for Community Services* (2006); *Independence, Well-being and Choice. Our Vision for the future of social care for adults in England* (2005b)) in which psychology has a key role to play.

Structure of this book

This book contains seven relatively short chapters that (hopefully) will engage you every step of the way. You will read, then stop and do some activities, discuss with colleagues (or friends, families, patients or the checkout operator at the local supermarket if you wish!), and then check your progress.

The book starts with **Chapter 1** (where better to start), a basic introduction to psychology – from a historical perspective (don't yawn – it is brief and relevant), through to the role of psychology across the lifespan and its role in healthcare – from cradle to grave. That means that the roles of psychology in pregnancy, in childhood, in adulthood and in old age and death are all highlighted. Finally, the social context of psychology and healthcare is explored, demonstrating the interplay between psychology, the social world and other disciplines.

In **Chapter 2**, the various schools of thought are presented. Being a relatively young science psychology has a number of 'schools of thought' or perspectives on how and why people behave in a certain manner. This chapter presents these various perspectives and highlights how they can be applied to your practice. Some of these perspectives will be useful for those working with children, other perspectives will be useful for those working with people with a learning difficulty or mental health issue and there will be other perspectives applicable across all nursing practices. However, be warned – this is a weighty chapter but it does provide an important overview of the various approaches adopted in psychology to explain how and why people behave.

Chapter 3 will explore psychology across the lifespan. It starts by exploring how psychologists have tried to explain the development of children from birth through to adolescence. It then explores how these developmental frameworks can be applied to nursing practice – whether this be at primary prevention level, dealing with mental heath issues or dealing with healthcare issues in the acute ward.

Chapter 4 looks at the social world – how we communicate with others through verbal and non-verbal means. It then looks at the power others have over us – conformity and obedience. Finally, we look at how these concepts and related issues can be put into practice when we introduce adherence to medical treatments.

The next chapter, **Chapter 5**, looks at cognitive psychology. It starts by exploring the concepts of perception and memory and how this can be related to nursing practice. The chapter then moves on from the 'pure' cognitive psychological areas and explores the social-cognition models of health behaviours and adherence (and the alternative forms of this term) to treatment. How these have been developed and how they can be used within practice to improve the care offered is explained.

Stress is the basis of **Chapter 6** – what it is, what causes it, what the consequences are. This is important from both a mental and physical health perspective as stress has the power to have negative consequences in a number of areas. The chapter finishes with some stress management techniques that are theory based – they are based on the models of stress presented earlier in the chapter.

The final chapter, **Chapter 7**, is the painful chapter. This chapter outlines the nature of pain, the models of pain and then how pain can be managed within a psychological framework. This is an application chapter (along with the stress chapter): you should be able to use your psychological knowledge and skills gathered from the previous chapters in these final two chapters.

Is this book for you?

This book is geared towards nursing students during their undergraduate studies, but it works equally well for those on post-graduate courses that require an additional psychological component. Students on any nursing branch will find the text useful, as will those on midwifery programmes. We also hope that practising nurses and other healthcare professionals will find this text valuable and a useful reference source.

Features of this book

We have tried to use a variety of pedagogical devices throughout this book with the intent of interesting the reader, reiterating the relevance of key points, and acting as a revision device.

Here are the special features in each chapter, designed to make you a better student:

LEARNING OUTCOMES

Each chapter starts with the sentence 'At the end of this chapter you will be able to'. This is to guide you and orientate you to what the chapter contains and what you can expect to have achieved by the end of the chapter.

YOUR STARTING POINT

A series of five multiple choice/short answer questions to test where you are starting from – these will be returned to later in the chapter.

KEY MESSAGE

A one sentence summary of the key message in a section.

QUICK CHECK

Asks you to recall or apply what you have just read. The answers can be found in the text and you should know the answer if you have read the text properly!

THINK ABOUT THIS

These ask the reader to consider a specific issue related to an individual topic under discussion. Obviously you can do this by yourself or with a colleague in order to increase your learning.

SUMMARY

At the end of each chapter we present a summary of the chapter in a series of bullet points. We hope that these will match the learning outcomes presented at the start of the chapter.

YOUR END POINT

Another series of questions for you to answer – if you have read the text, followed the exercises and discussed the issues then you should get them all correct.

FURTHER READING

We have included a few items that will provide additional information – some of these are in journals and some are full texts. For each we have provided the rationale for suggesting the additional reading and we hope that these will direct you accordingly.

WEBLINKS

A list of useful websites ends each chapter. We hope you will access these for further information.

REFERENCES

All the references cited throughout the text are gathered here. If you want to explore an area further then use these, along with the further reading suggestions, to expand your knowledge.

GLOSSARY

Finally, bold words in the text that may not be immediately familiar or are technical in nature are defined in the glossary.

WARNING

Finally, a warning for all readers. This text is written in a relaxed and informal style so that the key principles can be read, understood and appreciated easily. Hopefully, you will find the style appropriate so you will find the information and key principles relevant to your practice easy to digest. However, when writing your assignment, your research project, or even your journal article you should **NOT** copy the style of this text - you need to present your material in a formal academic style.

Beware of writing about tap dancing donkeys* in your formal academic reports!

---

*See Chapter 4.

Acknowledgements

This project, like all such projects, has been a major undertaking and one that (on more than one occasion) has felt more distant than it should have been. The production involved the assessment of range of sources – whether these be academic journal articles, internet sources or popular academic text books. This material then had to be digested into bite-sized, conversational pieces. I hope that I have done the researchers, clinicians and policy makers justice in the interpretation.

On a more personal level, several key colleagues have acted as researchers for us and have contributed their time, effort and opinions with vigour and a frankness that was as refreshing as it was useful. In particular I have to thank Stella Williamson, Erica Thomas, Alison Cartwright, Karen Policarpo and Charlotte Taylor. They all drafted a framework for individual chapters, contributed to the glossary or found references for this book and I am extremely grateful for the time and effort they put into the work. I am also thankful to Julia Mathias, my assistant at the University of Worcester, for keeping me (and all men) on the straight and narrow and dealing with the final details of this book.

Many thanks also to the team at Pearson publishing, in particular, Kate Brewin, for helping drive through this project. Her requests are asked so pleasantly and persuasively that I can never refuse – despite my initial resolution to be firm! Obviously, for a text like this the design is of key importance so thanks to all of those involved in the production of this text – the designers and production editors for enhancing the text with some excellent features, which we hope have provided guidance, direction and added value for all readers.

Finally, I must offer thanks and acknowledgements to those that have provided the support for us both at work and at home. For colleagues at the University of Worcester many thanks for your help, advice, friendship and practical guidance over the gestation period of this text.

Finally, I would like to thank my children – Rosie (my favourite), Francesca and Gabriel – for keeping out of the way, and Penney for not.

Publisher's acknowledgements

We are grateful to the following for permission to reproduce copyright material:

FIGURES

Figure 1.5 from Dahlgren, G and Whitehead, M, 1991, Stockholm Institute for Future Studies, *Policies and Strategies to Promote Social Equity in Health*.; Figure 5.12 from *Social Psychology and Health*, 2 ed., Open University Press (Stroebe. W 2000), Wolfgang Stroebe, *Social Psychology and Health*, 2000. Reproduced with the kind permission of Open University Press. All rights reserved.; Figure 5.13 from *Health Psychology: a textbook*, 3 ed., Open University Press (Ogden, J 2004), Jane Ogden, *Health Psychology*, 2004. Reproduced with the kind permission of Open University Press. All rights reserved.; Figure 7.6 from *Essentials of Pediatric Nursing*, 6, Elsevier (Wong, D.L 2001), From Hockenberry MJ, Wilson D, Wong's essentials of pediatric nursing, ed. 8, St. Louis, 2009, Mosby. Used with permission. Copyright Mosby.

TEXT

Box 3.1 from *Growing Old – Years of Fulfilment*, Addison Wesley (Kastenbaum, R 1979), KASTENBAUM, GROWING OLD, 1st Edition, (c) 1979. Reprinted by permission of Pearson Education, Inc., Upper Saddle River, NJ.

In some instances we have been unable to trace the owners of copyright material, and we would appreciate any information that would enable us to do so.

Chapter 1

Introduction: psychology in nursing care

LEARNING OUTCOMES

At the end of this chapter you will be able to:

- Understand the development of psychology as a science
- Appreciate some of the schools of thought in psychology
- Appreciate the research methods in psychology
- Understand the social context for health and health psychology
- Understand the role of psychology in many aspects of life
- Appreciate the role of psychology in all aspects of health and illness from the cradle to the grave.

YOUR STARTING POINT

Answer the following questions to assess your knowledge and understanding of the relationship between psychology and nursing and the key terms and principles underlying psychology.

1. By the 1920s a new definition of psychology had gained favour. Psychology was said to be the science of . . .

   (a) mind
   (b) consciousness
   (c) computers
   (d) behaviour
   (e) philosophy.

2. What is the independent variable, in experimental research?

   (a) a variable which nobody controls or changes
   (b) the variable which is manipulated in an experiment
   (c) the variable which is measured, to see results of an experiment
   (d) a variable which describes some durable characteristic of the subject
   (e) a variable which is held steady.

3. Cartesian dualism specifies that:

   (a) The body can interact with the mind via the pineal gland.
   (b) The mind can interact with the body via the pineal gland.
   (c) The mind and the body do not interact at all.
   (d) Both (a) and (b).
   (e) Neither (a) nor (b).

4. According to many, the founder of modern day psychology and first 'psychologist' was:

   (a) Wundt
   (b) Fechner
   (c) Weber
   (d) Helmholtz
   (e) None of the above.

5. Which of the following schools of thought would be most likely to reject the method of introspection to study human experience?

   (a) Behaviourism
   (b) Psychoanalysis
   (c) Structuralism
   (d) Functionalism
   (e) None of the above.

1.1 Introduction

Being a nurse is all about medicine and nursing practice, isn't it? It is all about bio-chemistry, physiology and anatomy? As a nurse you need to understand the patient's medical and nursing history, you need to understand their diagnosis and their treatment, you need to understand what is going on, inside the brain, the liver, the kidneys, the heart and so on. However, a human being is more than the sum of bodily parts (see Figure 1.1) and this has an important consequence for your nursing practice and the importance of psychology in healthcare.

It could be argued, of course, that your individual patient is not that concerned about their body parts – what they want is to get better in the shortest and most painless manner. They want to be treated with respect and dignity, they want to be

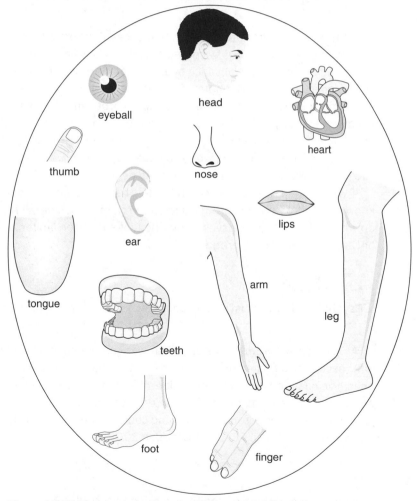

Figure 1.1 The human being is more than a sum of its parts

involved in their care and they want the nurse to act in a thoroughly professional manner. All of these have a psychological element.

KEY MESSAGE

Humans are more than a collection of organs.

The patient also wants to know what caused their illness – is there something that can be done about it, and if so, what? How can they prevent it from occurring again and how can they be included in their care? Again, all of these have a psychological element.

KEY MESSAGE

Psychology is the most important subject you will study.

We must also appreciate the definition of health as provided by the World Health Organisation (WHO, 1946): 'A complete state of physical, mental and social well-being and not merely the absence of disease or infirmity.' (I am sure that all readers will be able to recite this mantra if not at the start of their course, at least by the end!) This suggests that health is not simply a problem with the biochemistry, physiology or anatomy of the individual patient but that there is a contribution, and an equal one at that, of social and psychological factors to the state of health.

And now for a bit of controversy: overall, psychology will be the most important subject you will study during your nursing degree.

If we look at Table 1.1, we see on the left-hand side all the benefits that a good knowledge of psychology brings, and on the right-hand side, all the things you can do without knowledge of psychology. The table has been limited to just half a page because of space considerations.

KEY MESSAGE

Psychology is the most important topic known to humankind.

As you can see from the table (which was completed in a totally unbiased fashion), psychology has many perspectives that enable the student nurse (and, indeed, the qualified nurse) to appreciate the individuality and diversity of patients and clients. This is important in the construction and delivery of individualised care plans as stated throughout nursing courses and, of course The Code (Nursing and Midwifery Council's Code of Conduct, 2008).

QUICK CHECK

What is the definition of health according to the WHO?

Table 1.1 The role of psychology in nursing practice

The role of psychology in nursing practice	Where psychology is not involved in nursing practice
● Understanding of mental health issues ● Ability to communicate with peers ● Ability to communicate with patients and clients ● Ability to enhance adherence to treatment ● Ability to change maladaptive behaviour ● Ability to deal with the stresses and strains of practice ● Stress management ● Pain management ● Design of systems and operations in theatre, ITU and on the wards ● Ability to communicate with patients and clients irrespective of their needs, disability or health concern ● Understanding of human behaviour from cradle to grave	

So, what is psychology and what does it encompass? The word psychology means 'the study of the mind' (being made up of two Greek words – *psyche* – mind, soul or spirit and *logos* – knowledge, discourse or study). Many have subsequently defined psychology as the study of mind, behaviour, emotions and thought processes. It can assist us with understanding our patients and clients, but also ourselves.

The other definition that we should provide is 'health psychology'. This is, as the term suggests, how psychology can be applied to all aspects of health and the healthcare system – whether they be related to the aetiology of a particular condition, the treatment of a particular condition or the promotion of health in an individual's life. A longer, more formal definition is provided below.

Definition of health psychology

'Health psychology is the aggregate of the specific educational, scientific and professional contributions of the discipline of psychology to the promotion and maintenance of health, the prevention and treatment of illness, the identification of etiologic and diagnostic correlates of health, illness and related dysfunction, and the analysis and improvement of the health care system and health policy formation' (Matarazzo, 1982).

THINK ABOUT THIS

What do you consider the most important topic you are studying on your nursing course? Why?

QUICK CHECK

What is the definition of psychology and health psychology?

1.2 A brief history of psychology

Don't worry - this will not take long - however, there needs to be a brief overview of the development of psychology so you can appreciate its origins and hence its development within the nursing field. The schools of thought, or perspectives in psychology, that we will discuss in detail later in this book are indicated in Figure 1.2. However, the historical overview provides some information on those key figures that have been influential in psychology and how this relates to the current viewpoint and the perspectives that can be applied to healthcare.

The father of psychology is believed to be William Wundt, although he was originally a professor of physiology in Germany.

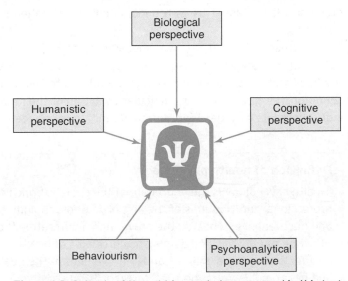

Figure 1.2 Schools of thought in psychology covered in this text

Wundt

Wundt wanted to apply the methodical, experimental methods of science to the study of human consciousness. To this end, he founded the first-ever psychology laboratory at the University of Leipzig in Germany in the 1880s. At his laboratory, Wundt spent hours exposing individuals to audio and visual stimuli and asking them to report what they perceived. In this way, he studied one component of consciousness, perception.

The school of thought that arose from the work of Wundt and his colleagues is called structuralism. The basic goal of structualists was to study consciousness by breaking it down into its components – mainly perception, sensation and affection. Their basic method was to train their subjects in introspection, which was careful, systematic observation of one's own conscious experience.

> **KEY MESSAGE**
> **Wundt believed in objective measurement – the initial scientific foundation of psychology.**

Structuralism vs. functionalism

An opposing school of thought – functionalism – was led by William James and John Dewey. While structuralists essentially wanted to determine 'what is consciousness?', functionalists wanted to determine 'what is consciousness used for?' – in other words, they wanted to study the purpose, or function, of consciousness and basic mental processes.

The two camps debated passionately over which approach to psychology was best, each hoping to shape the direction of their fledging academic subject. Although neither won the war, the creative tensions led to the establishment of the first psychology lab in the USA (Johns Hopkins University).

Behaviourism

Around 1913, American psychologist John B. Watson founded a new movement that changed the focus of psychology. He believed that internal mental processes should not be studied, because they cannot be observed; instead, Watson advocated that psychology focus on the study of behaviour and thus his movement became known as behaviourism. As Watson saw it, behaviour was not the result of internal mental processes, but rather the result of automatic response to stimuli from the environment. Behaviourism became focused on how conditions of the environment affect behaviour and, specifically, how humans learn new behaviour from the environment. This movement took a strong hold in America and was the dominant school of thought for about 40 years. Watson's successor, as the leader of behaviourism, was B.F. Skinner, who developed an influential view that operant conditioning was the mechanism for learning.

KEY MESSAGE

Behaviourism has played a significant part in mental health and learning disability nursing.

THINK ABOUT THIS

In the past day, think about a time you have given a reward (i.e. reinforced a behaviour). What about receiving a reward (i.e. reinforcer)? Has it made the behaviour more likely?

KEY MESSAGE

Behaviourism confines itself to the effect of the environment on behaviour.

Gestalt theory

While behaviourism was becoming dominant in the USA, two other schools gained influence in Europe around the same time. Gestalt theorists' basic belief was that any psychological phenomenon, from perceptual processes to human personality, should be studied holistically; that is, they should not be broken down into components, but rather studied as a whole.

Psychoanalysis

The second major movement in Europe at this time was psychoanalytic theory. This theory, developed by Austrian psychologist Sigmund Freud, revolutionised psychology and other aspects of modern thought. Very much the opposite of behaviourism, it focused on humans' internal workings and proposed a whole new way of explaining them. The theory developed by Freud was quite extensive and intricate, but the main principle is that the unconscious is responsible for most thought and behaviour in all people and the disorders of the mentally ill. Freud's psychoanalytic theory gained a wide following and many of his ideas are commonly believed by the public today. However, there is limited evidence and most psychologists consider Freud to be of interest merely from a historical perspective.

KEY MESSAGE

Psychology owes a lot to Freud, but his theory is now considered to have a limited evidence base and hence receives limited support.

THINK ABOUT THIS

Although Freud's theory is no longer considered valid, what value has his methods and theory still got in nursing practice?

Humanism

By the 1950s, a new movement began as an alternative to behaviourism and psychoanalytic theory. The followers of this movement considered behaviourism and psychoanalytic theory dehumanising and they took the name, humanism, for their movement. Instead of behaving as pawns of the environment or the powerful unconscious, humanists believed humans were inherently good and that their own mental processes played an active role in their behaviour. Free will, emotions and a subjective view of experience were important in the humanism movement.

Cognitive theory

The most recent major school of thought to arise has been the cognitive perspective, which began in the 1970s. This movement is much more objective and calculating than humanism, yet it is very different from behaviourism, as it focuses extensively on mental processes. The main idea of this movement is that humans take in information from their environment through their senses and then process the information mentally. The processing of information involves organising it, manipulating it, storing it in memory, and relating it to previously stored information. Cognitive theorists apply their ideas to language, memory, learning, dreams, perceptual systems and mental disorders.

Table 1.2 highlights how each of these areas is of central importance in psychology and in nursing practice and when they will be covered in the following chapters of this text.

QUICK CHECK

Who is the founder of modern psychology?

Which school of thought grew in opposition to the introspection approach?

1.3 The language of psychology

All subjects have their own special language – you will have come across some terms in nursing that you probably have not come across before. Just as it is in nursing, so it is in psychology. Psychology has its own jargon and it is probably

Table 1.2 Historical perspective on psychology's development

School of thought	Useful in nursing practice because . . .
Structuralism	Stressed the importance of scientific study of mental processes. An obvious link to mental health nursing and how psychological processes can impact on physical health (see Chapter 6).
Behaviourism	Emphasis was on the behaviour and how this could be influenced by the environment (see Chapter 2). Has a key role to play in working with children, people with learning disabilities, those with mental health issues and those in pain (i.e. many of the people nurses come across).
Gestalt	Importantly recognising that the human should be treated holistically and not as the sum of its individual parts (covered in Chapters 1 and 5).
Psychoanalysis	The importance of the unconscious was revealed and the link between psychological conflict and physical health was further highlighted (Chapter 2).
Humanism	The root of positive nursing practice.
Cognitive theory	The future (as some would see it) – a more scientific and information processing perspective that explores the way in which people make sense of their environment (see Chapter 2).

sensible that there is an introduction to this language before progressing any further. Psychology has its own terms including some words, phrases and approaches that may be familiar to you but mean different things to psychologists from normal (sic!) people.

For example, if a person says 'behaviour' then a psychologist would say 'define the behaviour'. If a person says 'personality' then a psychologist will ask 'which aspect of personality?'. Furthermore, psychologists from different traditions (see Table 1.2) would further refine the personality into an element that fits in with their understanding of the person. For example, a psychologist from the psychoanalytic tradition might suggest that a person has an 'anal expulsive personality' (stemming from the anal stage, a child who becomes fixated due to over-control transfers their unresolved anal/or control issues into characteristics such as cruelty, pushiness, messiness or disorganisation) or an 'anal retentive personality' (stemming from the anal stage, a child who becomes fixated due to under-control transfers their unresolved anal/or control issues into characteristics such as compulsivity, stinginess, cleanliness, organisation and obstinacy). These are phrases that will be uncommon to you (and probably to many psychologists as well) but they simply are there to demonstrate the point that individual psychologists speak a different language from other professions, and often, from each other.

There are, of course, many other such examples and it would be impossible to go through all of these – but you get the point! Psychologists have a language of their own, and this language may be further divided according to the psychologist's school of thought.

Having said that, however, there are a few terms that you should appreciate as being essential to the understanding of psychology. Firstly, psychology is a scientific discipline based on models, theory, hypotheses and empirical study.

> **THINK ABOUT THIS**
>
> List some terms you think of when thinking about psychology.

1.4 What is a science?

One common misconception about science is that it is all about statistics and hard maths! It is not – there are plenty of scientists that produced scientific theories without reaching for the calculator (think of Darwin or Piaget for example). Nor is science about technology – there are plenty of examples of technology that have no scientific basis (e.g. 'lie detector') and plenty of science that has no technology (e.g. Darwin once again). So, this is what science is not, but what are the central qualities of science and how does this relate to psychology?

> **KEY MESSAGE**
>
> Psychology is a science and uses scientific methods, language and approaches.

1.5 Key qualities of a science

All sciences share a common method of investigation: they are data driven and do not rely on personal biases or superstitions. This data is produced objectively and is subject to both replication by others and peer review. Hence, any study we conduct has to be clearly recorded and open to public scrutiny so it can be challenged and replicated. Furthermore, science examines solvable problems which are empirically derived and are not too all-encompassing (not looking for the meaning of life for example!). If we unpick this further, we see that for psychology to be defined as a science it has to have:

- **A defined subject matter:** we can clearly state the range of subject matter or phenomena that psychology studies.
- **Theory construction:** we can try to explain the observed phenomena in terms of theory (see Chapter 5 for how psychologists have attempted to do this).

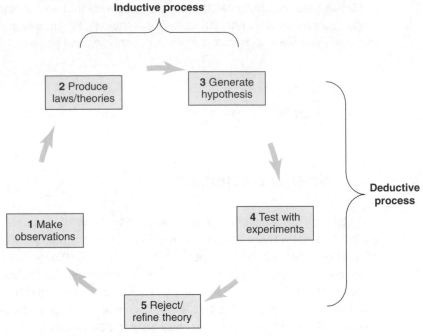

Figure 1.3 **The scientific method**

- **Hypothesis testing:** we can make specific predictions based on our theory which we can test empirically.
- **Empirical testing:** used to collect data (or evidence) to support or refute the hypothesis.

In Figure 1.3 the scientific induction-deduction method is outlined and shows how science progresses. At the first stage there is the inductive process, where psychologists (or other scientists) follow an inductive process where they observe instances of a natural phenomenon and derive a general law based on these observations. Hence, they are moving from the particular to the general. The next stage suggests that we move from the general to the particular - hence the theory has been derived and we now want to look for instances to confirm (or refute) our law or theories.

QUICK CHECK

List the central characteristics of a science.

Out of this perspective come a number of terms and methods that will crop up during this text:

- **Hypothetical constructs:** These are not observable but can only be inferred from behaviour. For example, memory, intelligence and personality.

- **Model:** A metaphor, involving a single fundamental idea or image.
- **Theory:** Often the terms theory and model are used, incorrectly, interchangeably, but a model is a complex set of inter-related statements that attempt to explain certain observed phenomena.
- **Hypothesis:** A testable statement about the relationship between two or more variables, based on a theory or model.
- **Variable:** Anything that can vary and can be one of two kinds: an independent variable (IV), which the researcher manipulates to see if it affects the dependent variable (DV).

One argument against psychology is that major sciences have paradigms, which are general theories that encompass many smaller theories. However, psychology does not have any of these. Instead, it has levels of explanations that are used to explain phenomena. Thomas Kuhn (Kuhn *et al.*, 1990) said that because of this 'psychology is a pre-science'. He meant that psychology had not quite reached the stage of being a science, but may do one day.

THINK ABOUT THIS

How would you define and measure the following:

- memory
- personality
- behaviour
- thinking?

1.6 Researching psychology

Psychology, as you would imagine, generates a considerable number of research questions and consequently requires a range of methods for gathering evidence to answer them. This text will not consider the whole gamut of research methods available, but will just skim the surface so you understand some of the terms that may come up in this text. There are a number of text books related to research methods and these can be accessed for further information when you need it.

Between groups design

A **between groups** design allocates matched groups of people to different treatments. If the measures are taken at one time this is a **cross-sectional design**, whereas if they are tested over two or more time periods then this would be a **longitudinal design**. For example, if we want to see whether a certain psychological approach (e.g. behavioural) to pain management works we would have one group that has the intervention (the experimental group) and another group (the control group) that does not. If we followed these people over time to see whether the behavioural intervention worked then it would be a longitudinal design.

We also have to remember to use an appropriate control group – we could not give the group nothing as the mere fact that the experimental group were receiving the intervention might be enough to cause improvement. So, we have to include a **placebo** control as treatment. This might be a non-specific treatment that does not involve the behavioural intervention.

Within participants design

This type of design is used when the same people provide measures at more than one time and differences between the measures at the different times are recorded. An example would be a measure taken before an intervention and again after the intervention. For example, you introduce a psychological intervention to try to improve the mental health of a group of people with learning disabilities living in supported accommodation. You measure the levels of mental health before the treatment, and then again after you have undertaken the intervention. There are obvious problems with this – did we keep everything else constant? How can you be sure that it was to down to the intervention specifically?

QUICK CHECK

List the advantages and disadvantages of a between participants and within participants design.

Cross-sectional studies

These studies obtain the responses from a group of participants on one occasion only. With appropriate randomised sampling methods, the sample can be assumed to be a representative cross-section of the population under study. So, for example, we can explore how many people are under stress at any one point in time. If we collect enough participants then we can probably also compare specific subgroups: is stress greater in men than women, is it greater in nurses or doctors (or psychologists)? These studies are quite common, but we must make sure the sample is representative and we cannot infer any cause and effect.

Observations

A simple kind of study involves observing behaviour in a relevant setting. Hence, we can explore interactions within a consultation setting: how do patients react to bad news? How do nurses react to giving good news?

Structured interviews

An interview schedule is prepared with a standard set of questions that are asked of each person, by telephone or by face-to-face interview. A semi-structured interview is more open ended and allows the interviewee to address issues that they feel are relevant to the interview.

Longitudinal design

These designs involve measuring responses of a single sample on more than one occasion over a period of time. These can either be prospective (where the recordings are taken and then planned for the future) or retrospective (where the recordings are obtained from already collected records). These types of designs are among the most powerful designs available for the evaluation of treatment and of theories about human behaviour.

Meta-analysis

This is a statistical analysis of the results from a number of studies already completed. A useful definition was given by Huque (1988): 'A statistical analysis that combines or integrates the results of several independent clinical trials considered by the analyst to be "combinable".'

Questionnaires

This is a popular and frequently employed method of study in psychology. Questionnaires consist of a standard set of items with accompanying instructions. Ideally a questionnaire will be both reliable (i.e. measure the same thing on more than one occasion) and valid (i.e. measure the thing that they say they are measuring). Questionnaires can be designed specifically for the study under discussion or they can be picked 'off the shelf' since many have already been designed (see Bowling (1995) for further details).

Surveys

This is a systematic method for determining how a sample of participants respond to a set of questions (or questionnaires) at one or more times. For example, we may want to know what people with alcohol problems think of the service they are receiving and how this compares to the views of the service providers. In this case we would do two surveys - one with the service users, and one with the service providers.

Randomised controlled trials

Randomised controlled trials (RCTs) involve the systematic comparison of interventions using a fully controlled application of one or more 'treatments' with a random allocation of participants to the different treatment groups. This design is the 'gold standard' to which much research in psychology and healthcare aspires. People are allocated at random (by chance alone) to receive one of several interventions. One of these interventions is the standard of comparison or control. The control may be a standard practice, a placebo or no intervention at all. RCTs seek to measure and compare the outcomes after the participants receive the interventions.

THINK ABOUT THIS

What design would you use to investigate whether:

- a behavioural approach to pain management worked in older people;
- painting the walls blue increased the quality of life in a children's ward;
- people with a learning disability in supported housing had better language skills than when living within their families;
- stress causes mental health problems;
- 'hard' drug users have a different personality to non-drug users.

What methodological and ethical considerations should you take into account?

Qualitative techniques

The methods discussed so far are quantitative techniques favoured by many in psychology and healthcare. However, there are also a number of qualitative techniques that may be of use. For example, there are **diary studies** which can help the researcher collect information about the temporal changes in health status (e.g. dealing with a life limiting condition). There are also narrative approaches in which the desire is to seek insight and meaning about health and illness through the acquisition of data in the form of stories concerning personal experiences (e.g. dealing with substance abuse). **Cases studies** provide a 'thick description' of a phenomenon that would not be obtained by the usual quantitative or qualitative approach. **Focus groups** are a common approach which involves a group of participants discussing a focused question or topic which can lead to the generation of interactive data.

KEY MESSAGE

Qualitative and quantitative techniques are both useful and valid techniques. You must use the most appropriate method for your research question.

Action research

Action research is increasingly being used within health, nursing and psychology and has been recommended by the Department of Health as a valuable approach for public health research (DoH, 2001). At its heart is the idea of using research to directly change practice. While other quantitative and qualitative research approaches may go through a long process of data collection, analysis and eventually producing a final report which researchers can only hope practitioners will use to inform their work, action research works directly with practitioners or community members so that findings are used immediately and continually to develop practice. Hence, a core idea within action research is that it is done *with* participants rather than *on* them. Lewin, who is considered the founder of action research, suggests that it 'proceeds in a spiral of steps each of which is composed of a circle of planning, action and fact-finding about the result of the action' (Lewin, 1946: 15).

This basic principle of a spiral of steps lives on in the design of many action research studies. A simple diagram of the action research spiral is shown in Figure 1.4.

Many action research studies now aim to empower the disempowered and to challenge the social structures that create such power imbalances. These developments have led to what has become known as 'participatory action research'. Participatory action research is built on the concept of a group of co-researchers working together as equal participants trying out various actions, evaluating and reflecting on their effectiveness as a group and then developing and, hopefully, improving their actions. Through this process the co-researchers begin not only to analyse the situation they are in, but also to build a sense of empowerment as they are able to take action to respond to their analysis.

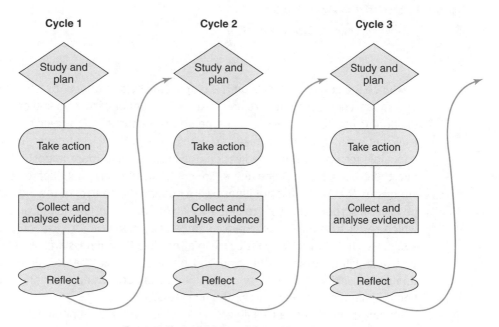

Progressive problem solving with action research

Figure 1.4 The action research spiral

> **KEY MESSAGE**
>
> Action research is a useful technique for involving users in research in order to improve services.

1.7 Health and health psychology in a social world

The definitions of health and illness can be the subject of a book themselves – indeed many texts have been written on this subject. However, for the purposes of this book we will use the definition of health provided by the World Health Organisation (1946):

> 'Health is a state of complete physical, mental and social well-being and not merely the absence of disease or infirmity.'

We will use this definition not necessarily because it is the best one, but because it is the one that all of us know and that many people cite. Despite its flaws (e.g. it is too idealistic) it does provide a good basis for future study and aspirational care. What this does suggest is that health is not merely about bugs, germs, accidents or biochemistry – it is about social and psychological variables as well.

> **THINK ABOUT THIS**
>
> How else can you define health?

Hence the current focus is on the **biopsychosocial** model of health and illness. This model considers illness to be a result of a number of factors and hence the individual is not seen as passive: the person can contribute to their health and to their ill-health. The person takes an active role in their treatment – they are responsible for taking their medication, for example, and more importantly changing their beliefs and behaviours. In contrast, the original biomedical model suggested that the causes of illness were outside the control of the individual – all physical disorders can be explained by disturbances in physiological processes, which result from injury, biochemical imbalance, bacterial or viral infections and so on. Psychology had very little role in either health or illness and no relationship was postulated between the mind and physical illness (the so-called **Cartesian dualism**). Luckily most people have come to their senses and recognise that psychology has a role to play in health and illness!

If we explore what causes illness from a biopsychosocial perspective then it is not simply a case of looking for a biological causative agent or physiological or genetic marker, we have to look additionally at both social and psychological factors.

Bio	Psycho	Social
Viruses	Behaviour	Class
Bacteria	Beliefs	Gender
Genetics	Stress	Ethnicity

Biological factors are, perhaps, more apparent and include such factors as the genetic make-up of the individual along with anatomy, physiology and chemical balance. Illness is caused by involuntary physical changes caused by such factors as chemical imbalance, bacteria, viruses and genetic predisposition.

Psychological factors include such variables as lifestyle (e.g. smoking, drinking) along with personality. It also includes such variables as cognition – thinking and interpreting, and beliefs. Emotional factors are also important in determining whether we seek out medical or some other form of healthcare assistance. Motivational factors are another factor under the psychological variable: if we are motivated when we start an exercise programme we are more likely to keep up with the programme.

QUICK CHECK

What is Cartesian dualism and how does it relate to healthcare?

Social factors are both broad and deep. All of us live in a social world – we all have relationships with others, whether these be our family, our friends or our work colleagues. Children may start smoking if their peer group encourages it because it may make them feel more grown up. These may be referred to as social norms of behaviour (whether it is OK to smoke or thought 'cool' to drink to excess) and relate to social values on health.

THINK ABOUT THIS

Consider an individual that comes to you with one of the following diagnoses:

- myocardial infarction/heart attack
- schizophrenia
- hepatitis
- kidney stones
- depression
- alcohol abuse.

What biological, psychological and social factors could be implicated? Is any one of the factors alone sufficient?

Now consider how you would treat them. What intervention would you suggest? How would you employ psychological and social variables?

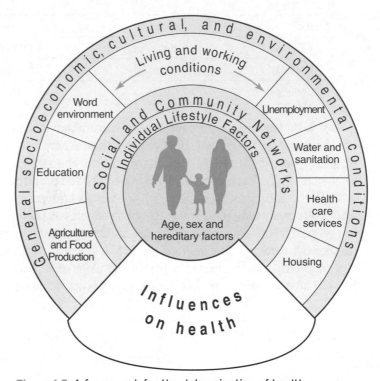

Figure 1.5 **A framework for the determination of health**

Source: Dahlgren, G. and Whitehead, M. (1991) *Policies and Strategies to Promote Social Equity in Health,* Stockholm, Sweden: Institute for Futures Studies.

The role of social factors in health, illness and psychology is of paramount importance. In Figure 1.5, an example framework for considering the general determinants of health is presented. The framework is multi-layered like an onion with the fixed factors at the core over which we have no control (e.g. age, sex and genetic factors) but surrounded by four layers of influence that we can do something about, either through psychological or social change.

This is a useful framework for understanding health and illness and the role of psychology within it. As Marks (2005) points out, the framework has six positive characteristics:

● It is concerned with all of the determinants of health, not simply with the course of events during the treatment of illness.

● It places the individual at the core but acknowledges the primary determining influence of society through the community, living and working conditions, and the surrounding socio-economic, cultural and environmental conditions.

● It places each layer in the context of its neighbours, reflecting the whole situation including possible structural constraints upon change.

● It has a true interdisciplinary flavour and is not purely a medical or quasi-medical model of health.

- It is even-handed and makes no claims for any one discipline as being more important than others.
- It acknowledges the complex nature of health determinants.

THINK ABOUT THIS

In light of the framework of Dahlgren and Whitehead (1991), what factors would you consider to be involved in the following:

- myocardial infarction/heart attack;
- schizophrenia;
- hepatitis;
- kidney stones
- depression
- alcohol abuse?

This means that we have to be aware of the socio-cultural variables and their potential impact on both psychology and health. We should be aware of the following broad factors:

- **Gender:** in industrialised societies today men die younger than women, yet women have poorer health than men. Men tend to die, on average, 6–8 years younger than their female counterparts. However, women have higher morbidity rates – women suffer more chronic and acute illnesses than men, and visit and spend more time in the hospital. Psychosocial and lifestyle differences account for many of these differences.

- **Ethnicity:** evidence suggests that the health of minority ethnic groups is generally poorer than that of the majority population. This pattern has been consistently observed in the USA and the UK. There are many possible explanations for these health differences. For example, racism means that minority ethnic groups are the subject of discrimination at a number of different levels. Secondly, ethnocentrism in health services, health promotion and access to health services favours the needs of the majority population. Finally, there are cultural differences and these may be highlighted in health protective behaviours and health damaging behaviours.

- **Socio-economic status (SES):** evidence from many studies over many years has indicated that there is a strong and consistent relationship between SES (or social class) and health. Specifically, the data suggests continuously increasing poor health as SES changes from high to low. The mediators of SES effects on health experience are likely to be behavioural and psychosocial. The behavioural factors include diet, exercise and smoking while the psychosocial factors include such processes as self-efficacy, self-esteem and perceived control (Siegrist and Marmot, 2004).

THINK ABOUT THIS

When treating or interacting with a patient, what psychosocial variables must you take into account?

KEY MESSAGE

Psychology as applied to health cannot be taken in isolation – you have to take note of the cultural context.

QUICK CHECK

What are the layers on the Dahlgren and Whitehead (1991) model? Why is this model of value?

1.8 The scope of psychology

Psychology has strong links with a range of other disciplines. At one end of the spectrum we have sociology and social anthropology – exploring societies and communities. This can be linked to social psychology and, as we will see during this chapter, the link to health and health psychology is also strong. One example is stress and social support. We get considerable support from our social relationships and this can be of benefit both psychologically and physically. As we will see in Chapter 4, the benefits derived from social networks can be considerable and can reduce the impact of stress and thereby improve health and well-being.

At the other end of the psychological spectrum we have the biological basis of our actions and activities. For example, when we look at pain in Chapter 7 we note that pain is a both a psychological and a biological construct: both of these factors are central to our understanding of pain and, consequently, to its management (see Figure 1.6 for an indication of the scope of psychology and its links across to other disciplines).

THINK ABOUT THIS

What other disciplines can psychology and nursing link with? Expand the diagram.

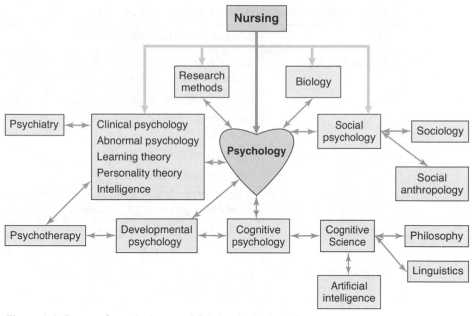

Figure 1.6 Scope of psychology and link to other disciplines

1.9 Psychology in health and nursing care

Given the nature of psychology and its links with a considerable number of other disciplines it will come as no surprise that psychology has a central role in health and illness. Consequently, when exploring psychological links to health, illness and healthcare, we find that at every step of the journey there is a role for psychology both through an untroubled life (see Table 1.3) and if there was an ill-health episode (see Table 1.4).

Table 1.3 Psychology's involvement across the lifespan

Event	Example of psychology's input
Conception ↓	Psychology can assist with family planning to ensure that either safe sex is practised (or isn't in the case of conception!) and that the psychological and physical states are maximised for the developing foetus (e.g. behaviour change to maximise health state).
Pregnancy ↓	Behaviour change to enhance health states (e.g. stop smoking sessions).
Labour and birth ↓	Social support reduces time in labour and pain associated with it.

(Continued)

Table 1.3 Psychology's involvement across the lifespan (*Continued*)

Event	Example of psychology's input
Child growing up ↓	Appreciation of the cognitive stage of development and the impact this has on understanding of health and illness.
Adolescence ↓	Potential optimum time to develop positive health behaviours. Mental health difficulties may appear – interventions required.
Adulthood ↓	Enhancing health behaviours. Changing health behaviours. Support for any maladaptive psychological or physical ill-health.
Late adulthood ↓	Coping with physical and cognitive decline. Support and methods for dealing with potential social isolation.
Death and bereavement	Support through bereavement, dealing with grief and preparing for death.

Table 1.4 Examples of role of psychology during health and illness

Stage	Example of psychology's input
Person is healthy ↓	Maintaining health. Promoting healthy behaviours. Reducing stress and promoting mental health. Reducing inappropriate health behaviours.
Person feels ill ↓	How does a person become aware of symptoms? How does a person respond to sensations? How does a person perceive that they are unwell? How does a person interpret symptoms?
Plans to visit healthcare professional ↓	Why does a person make the choice to go to the healthcare professional at that time? What prompts (or who prompts) the person to go? How does the person respond to symptoms? What is the role of family and friends in deciding to visit the healthcare professional?
Visits healthcare professional ↓	What does the person tell the healthcare professional? How does the person communicate (both verbally and non-verbally) in the consultation? What are the factors that influence the consultation? How does the healthcare professional react? What cognitive processing does the healthcare professional go through to reach their conclusion?

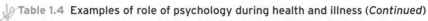

Table 1.4 Examples of role of psychology during health and illness (*Continued*)

Stage	Example of psychology's input
Diagnosis and treatment ↓	How does the healthcare professional come to their diagnosis and choice of treatment?
	How does the patient react to the diagnosis?
	How does the patient react to the treatment plan?
	How does the person react to becoming a patient?
	Is the person satisfied with the consultation?
	Did they understand and remember the diagnosis and treatment?
Living with an illness ↓	How does living with an illness affect the self?
	How has the illness affected the individual's quality of life?
	What impact does the diagnosis have on family and friends?
	What is the role of family and friends in dealing with the diagnosis and illness?
	How does the illness affect the emotions of the person?
	How does the family and individual adjust to the diagnosis?
Dealing with pain ↓	What is pain?
	How can pain be affected by the illness and the reaction to the illness?
	What is the role of the family in managing pain?
	How does pain influence quality of life?
Coming to the end of life ↓	What stages does the person go through on diagnosis?
	How can the healthcare practitioner help the person come to terms with their impending death?
	How can the family and friends be supported?

Both of these are rather extreme examples, going from a perfectly fit person through to a dead person within a few steps. However, they are there to serve a point: psychology plays an important role in our lives, whether we be healthy or ill, whether we are young or old, or whether we are at the start of our life or at the end of it.

1.10 Conclusion

This book has been designed to provide you with the insight you need to demonstrate how important psychology is to your professional role. Whilst not all of the topics highlighted in Tables 1.3 and 1.4 are covered in this text, there is enough information here for you to find useful and informative, and to help move your professional career forward.

1.11 Summary

- Psychology has an important role to play in nursing.
- The WHO definition of health encompasses both biological and psychosocial elements.
- Psychology is the study of the mind and behaviour.
- Psychology has its origins in the systematic, experimental study of human consciousness.
- Psychology has its own language and terminology.
- Psychology is a science and employs a number of methods in order to complete research studies.
- Action research is a useful technique for involving users in research in order to improve services.
- The role of psychosocial factors should not be overlooked.
- Psychology has links with a number of other disciplines.
- Psychology has a role across the lifespan both in health and in illness.

YOUR END POINT

Answer the following questions to assess your knowledge and understanding of the relationship between psychology and nursing and the key terms and principles underlying psychology.

1. The cognitive revolution in psychology was a response to the limitations of which school of thought?
   (a) Psychoanalysis
   (b) Behaviourism
   (c) Human information-processing
   (d) Gestalt psychology
   (e) All of the above.

2. Psychologists employ a variety of tools and methods to study human behaviour. Which of the following methods do psychologists rely on to make systematic observations and draw conclusions about human behaviour?
   (a) Speculation and common sense
   (b) Generalisation and common sense
   (c) Hindsight and experimentation
   (d) Controlled measurement and experimentation
   (e) Personal experience and collective wisdom.

3. The study of psychology is most concerned with which field of scientific inquiry?

(a) The science of philosophy
(b) The science of behaviour and mental processes
(c) The science of developmental processes
(d) The science of physical processes
(e) The science of emotional and mental processes.

4. Which of the following might affect an individual's view about issues in psychology?

(a) Socio-cultural context
(b) Political beliefs
(c) Sources of funding
(d) All of the above
(e) None of the above.

5. What is the main focus of the nature/nurture debate in psychology?

(a) Child development
(b) Gender difference research
(c) Race difference research
(d) Personality and intelligence
(e) None of the above.

Further reading

Angoff, W.H. (1988). The nature–nurture debate, aptitudes and group differences. *American Psychologist*, 43, pp. 713-720.

Eysenck, M.W. (2000). *Simply Psychology*. Hove, UK: Psychology Press.

Fischer, C.T. (2006). *Qualitative Research Methods in Psychology: Introduction through Empirical Studies*. Boston: Academic Press.

Fisher, S. and Greenberg, R.P. (1996). *Freud Scientifically Reappraised: Testing the Theories and Therapy*. Chichester, UK: Wiley.

Gravetter, F.J. and Forzano, L.A.B. (2002). *Research Methods for the Behavioural Sciences*. New York: Thompson/Wadworth.

Kimble, G.A., Wertheimer, M. and White, C.L. (1991). *Portraits of Pioneers in Psychology*. Washington, DC: American Psychological Association and Hillsdale, NJ: Lawrence Erlbaum Associates.

Whitehead, D. (2001). Health education, behavioural change and social psychology: Nursing's contribution to health promotion? *Journal of Advanced Nursing*, 34(6), pp. 822-832.

Weblinks

http://www.behavenet.com
Behavioural Health Care Information. This site contains all the latest news and developments in behavioural healthcare. There are also links to the latest behavioural healthcare articles.

http://www.onlinepsychresearch.co.uk
Online Psychology Research. This site actually gives you the chance to take part in real psychology studies online. Make a contribution to psychological knowledge today.

http://www.behavior-analyst-online.org
Behaviour Analyst Online. This site contains links to behaviour analysis journals.

http://www.all-about-psychology.com
All about Psychology. This site, as the name suggests, is all about psychology. It contains definitions, history, topic areas, theory and practice.

http://www.dcity.org/braingames/stroop/index.htm
Stroop Test Demonstration. This site allows you to take part in a classic psychology test. The test demonstrates the difficulties we can all have in processing information. Have a go!

Chapter 2

Psychological approaches to understanding people

LEARNING OUTCOMES

At the end of this chapter you will be able to:

- Name and explain at least four approaches in psychology to understanding the person

- Understand the psychoanalytical approach to understanding the person

- Appreciate the concepts, terminology and approach of the behavioural explanation

- Develop the cognitive approach to the person and how this can be applied to nursing and healthcare

- Explain how social learning theory has been applied to understanding the person

- Understand the humanistic approach to the person

- Express the ideas of major theorists within each approach

- Evaluate each approach in terms of its strengths and weaknesses

- Demonstrate the application of each approach to nursing and health practice.

YOUR STARTING POINT

Answer the following questions to assess your knowledge and understanding of the psychological approaches to understanding the person.

1. Some of the areas involved in psychology are:

   (a) psychoanalytic theory
   (b) behaviourism
   (c) cognitive psychology
   (d) social learning theory
   (e) all of the above.

2. According to psychoanalytic theory:

   (a) All behaviour is learned.
   (b) Behaviour is the result of maladaptive thinking.
   (c) Behaviour is the result of physiological processes.
   (d) Behaviour is the result of innate drives and early experiences.
   (e) Behaviour is the result of vicarious reinforcement.

3. Behaviourism is concerned with:

   (a) unobservable mental states
   (b) modelling
   (c) defence mechanisms
   (d) observable behaviour
   (e) none of the above.

4. According to the information processing approach:

   (a) The mind is analogous to a computer.
   (b) It doesn't matter what goes on inside the 'black box'.
   (c) Culture plays a major role in cognitive development.
   (d) Thinking is information processing.
   (e) (a) and (d).

5. Social learning theory is concerned with:

   (a) cognition
   (b) observation
   (c) modelling
   (d) vicarious reinforcement
   (e) all of the above.

2.1 How psychology helps us to understand why people do what they do

Why do people do what they do? Why do people behave in a certain way? Why is it that some people leave their assignment to the day before it is due in, whilst others do it in an organised and systematic manner? Why is it that certain individuals are aggressive and outspoken, and others patient and understanding? Why is it that certain people want to become nurses, whereas others want to become psychologists or physiotherapists? Why is it that certain nurses enjoy working with older people, whereas others enjoy working with children? These sorts of questions have been addressed by psychologists in a range of different ways to formulate approaches to explaining the person.

An approach is a perspective (i.e. view) that involves certain beliefs about people and the way that they function. There maybe several different theories within each approach, but they all share some common underlying assumptions. Unfortunately (or fortunately depending on your perspective), there are several different approaches in psychology and there are many reasons for this. Firstly, it is because all psychologists argue with each other and enjoy this experience! There is no real agreed position, and there may be several factors that influence the way we behave – there is no conclusive evidence for any one of the approaches.

However, the most important reason for different approaches existing is because our behaviour is determined by several factors: for example our genetic endowment, physiological processes, personal characteristics such as intelligence, personality and **psychopathology**, the environment, specific stimuli and cognitive processes such as perception, thoughts, memories and so on.

THINK ABOUT THIS

Why do people act in this way:

- yawn
- eat too much
- drink alcohol
- are short tempered
- don't follow your advice
- get depressed
- have phobias about spiders, needles or uniforms?

The idea that there are various explanations for human behaviour can be illustrated by taking a concrete example. For example, most people now agree that substance abuse and substance dependence are determined by a range of factors: 'a multiply determined phenomena' (Lowe, 1995).

> **THINK ABOUT THIS**
>
> Think about all the factors associated with substance misuse. List them all. Is there any way you can categorise them, into social, biological and so on?

When we have listed all the factors associated with substance misuse we may come up with variables such as social factors (e.g. stressful living conditions or unemployment) or you may suggest some biological factors (such as the genes the individual inherited from their parents). You may also come up with other suggestions – personality characteristics which make the individual prone to substance abuse or the reduction in tension and raised spirits that substance use may bring about (which could be broadly described as psychological factors). Indeed all of the variables you listed may simultaneously contribute to substance abuse/dependency behaviours. So no clear answer there then!

Of course, human behaviour is so complex that it cannot be understood simply by one approach; we have to accept the inevitable – it is multi-faceted. Just as trying to explain a complex behaviour like substance misuse is confusing, so is trying to understand relatively simple behaviours such as arriving early or late for appointments or food preference.

In this chapter we introduce key psychological approaches to explaining behaviour and how we can apply them to your nursing practice. Firstly, we overview the basic ideas behind the psychodynamic approach before looking at how the shortcomings of these ideas led to behaviourism. We will then go on to examine social learning theory, which attempts to extend behaviourist ideas, before finally considering the cognitive approach.

> **KEY MESSAGE**
>
> Attempting to understand the person by just one psychological perspective is impossible.

2.2 The psychodynamic approach

The term 'psychodynamic' refers to a collection of theories that try to account for the dynamics of human behaviour; 'dynamics' are the things that drive us or motivate us to behave in particular ways. The **psychodynamic approach** explores how the mind (especially the unconscious mind) is responsible for everyday behaviour. The most influential psychodynamic theorist is Sigmund Freud (1856–1939) and he will be the main focus of this section.

Freud was a medical doctor in Austria and became interested in how the 'mind' could influence physical symptoms of the body. Freud began to experiment with **hypnosis**, but soon found that its beneficial effects were short-lived. At this point he decided to adopt a method suggested by his colleague and close friend Josef Breuer, which later came to be known as the **talking cure**. Breuer had discovered that when he encouraged his neurotic patients to talk openly about the earliest experiences of their symptoms, their symptoms gradually subsided. In collaboration with Breuer, Freud developed the idea that many **neuroses** (e.g. phobias, paranoia, hysterical paralyses and pain) had their origins in traumatic events experienced in childhood but which were now forgotten. The belief that all behaviour originates from childhood experiences that reside within the unconscious is called **psychic determinism**.

> **KEY MESSAGE**
> Psychoanalysis highlights the importance of unconscious drives.

> **Basic assumptions behind the psychodynamic approach**
> - Much of our behaviour is determined by unconscious thoughts and desires.
> - Maladaptive behaviour is the result of unresolved unconscious conflicts originating in childhood.
> - Resolution occurs through accessing and confronting unresolved conflicts.

2.3 Psychoanalytic theory

Freud's psychoanalytic theory seeks to explain behaviour in terms of an interaction between innate drives (i.e. those we were born with and which we all have) and early experiences in childhood. In order to fully understand Freud's theory and its application to your practice, we first need to explain some important concepts: Freud's topography and structure of the mind; defence mechanisms; the theory of infantile sexuality and the Oedipus complex.

Freud's topography of mind

According to Freud, the mind has three levels: the **conscious, pre-conscious** and **unconscious**. The conscious part of the mind deals with the here and now. The pre-conscious part of the mind contains feelings, thoughts and experiences from

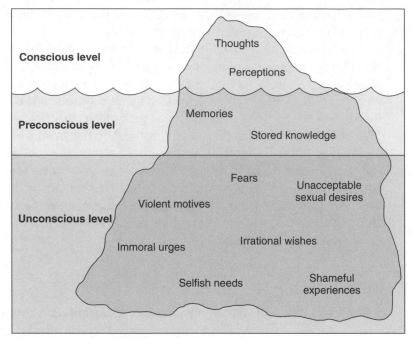

Figure 2.1 Freud's analogy for the human mind

the past that could easily be retrieved from memory and brought back to conscious awareness. The unconscious part of the mind contains information that the individual is not consciously aware of; this information is very hard and sometimes impossible to retrieve. Freud often used an iceberg analogy (see Figure 2.1) to illustrate the amount of importance given to the unconscious. Just as the major portion of an iceberg lies below the water's surface, a major portion of the human psyche lies below the level of awareness. Freud believed that causal factors responsible for human behaviour reside at this level of the mind. Therefore to understand human behaviour, the unconscious must be revealed.

Freud's topography of mind forms the main premise of **psychoanalysis**. Psychoanalysis is a form of therapy which aims to help the patient gain deeper insight into their behaviour by exploring their unconscious thoughts and emotions. Although nurses cannot practise psychoanalysis unless they are fully trained, the principles of this approach may be useful in situations where the cause of a patient's complaint is not apparent and may warrant further exploration.

Freud's structural model of the mind

Freud also assumed that the mind could be divided into three basic sections; the **id, ego** and **superego**. This constitutes Freud's structural model of the mind and can be said to represent impulsivity, rationality and morality respectively. The id is the part of the mind which contains innate sexual (libido) and aggressive instincts and is located in the unconscious. The id is based on the 'pleasure principle' which drives the desire for immediate satisfaction.

The second component of the mind is the superego, which contains the morals and rules of society. The superego develops as a result of the Oedipus complex (which will be discussed below) and usually emerges between the ages of three and six years. The main purpose of the superego is to prevent gratification of the id's desires by observing the rules and regulations that operate within society.

Finally, the third component of the mind is the ego. The ego is based on the 'reality principle' and mediates between the id's innate desires and the moral standards of the superego. An important part of Freud's theory was the notion that there are frequent conflicts among the id, ego and superego, which cause the individual to experience anxiety. Consequently the ego devotes much time to trying to resolve these conflicts with the use of ego defence mechanisms.

QUICK CHECK

What are the components of the mind according to Freud?

QUICK CHECK

We can try to apply the concepts of id, ego, superego by looking for manifestations or representations of each of these concepts in some text or aspect of life. For example, in *Sex and the City* we may get:

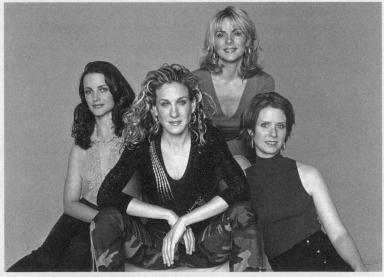

| Charlotte (Superego) | Carrie (Id) | Miranda (Ego) |

Now you try to find characters that fit into each of these concepts:

Topic	Id (emotion)	Ego (pure rationality)	Superego (command)
Books			
Films			
Heroes/heroines			
Songs			
TV programmes			
Your work colleagues			
Your student peers			
Your patients			

Ego defence mechanisms

The ego protects itself by employing a number of **defence mechanisms**. According to Hough (2002), defence mechanisms are strategies designed to protect the individual against painful anxiety and ensure that the ego is not overwhelmed. Over a dozen defence mechanisms have been proposed by Freud and his followers. Among those commonly described are displacement, sublimation, projection, reaction formation, rationalisation and denial. The most basic and fundamental defence mechanism is called **repression** and implies the purposeful forgetting of anxiety-laden thoughts, memories or desires. Extreme reactions as well as high levels of anxiety can be indicative of repressed thoughts and feelings. In order to resolve these issues, the patient or client should be invited to talk about their anxieties and encouraged to discharge negative emotions, thoughts, memories and so on. This is referred to as **catharsis** (although please note that specialist education is required to practise psychoanalysis properly).

Displacement – often referred to as 'kick the cat syndrome' – involves the expression of an unconscious impulse, but against a substitute person, animal or object. If a displacement results in some socially acceptable or beneficial activity it is called **sublimation.** In recent years there have been several highly publicised cases in which carers have neglected or mistreated elderly patients. One possible Freudian explanation for this unacceptable behaviour is displacement. For example, research suggests that the stress of caring is often identified as a trigger for elder abuse (Wieland, 2000), although this has not always been found (e.g. Action on Elder Abuse, 2004).

Projection is a defence mechanism which involves getting rid of one's own undesirable characteristics by attributing them to others. The person who is projecting may accuse others of hating them or wishing them harm, when actually they are the one guilty of these thoughts and emotions. For instance, a patient who dislikes a nurse could project by openly accusing the nurse of being unfriendly or hostile. Nurses need to be aware of projection and, if such a situation arises, not take the feelings of the patient personally.

In **reaction formation**, an anxiety-laden impulse, thought or feeling is replaced in consciousness by its opposite. Loss of control, self-esteem and/or self-worth can result in the patient concealing such feelings and instead portraying a blasé, over-confident or even aggressive façade. In fact Ferns (2007) found that factors such as pain, fear and anxiety were closely linked to aggression in acute care settings. In **denial** the ego is incapable of dealing with threatening facts and therefore fails to acknowledge the reality of this information. Aligned with health practice, denial can manifest itself as a mechanism for denying the presence of illness and medical diagnoses (Kreitler, 1999). Denial itself can be healthy to a certain extent and is part of the normal coping process featured within many of the grief framework models (Rana and Upton, 2009). However, denial can become problematic when it interferes with compliance with medical advice or ongoing treatment. Research suggests that nurses should work with rather than confront patient denial. According to Houldin (2000), direct confrontation of patient denial will only result in the increased use of this defence mechanism, therefore it is better to support the patient and discuss issues of concern which they will be able to think about at their own pace.

Finally, **regression** is another type of defence mechanism which is closely linked to **fixation** and the theory of infantile sexuality which will be discussed next. In regression, during times of stress, individuals will retreat to behaviours which are comforting and characteristic of an earlier stage of development. For example, an individual who is diagnosed with cancer may seek comfort and thus retreat to a childhood state by rocking backwards and forwards. Displaying regression should indicate to the nurse that the patient is anxious and coping by comforting themselves. Nurses should aim to reduce patient anxiety by offering appropriate information and coping strategies which encourage relaxation. Defence mechanisms are indicative of high levels of anxiety. A nurse who is familiar with defence mechanisms can help the patient move forward psychologically by tailoring communication to encourage and facilitate catharsis.

QUICK CHECK

List the ego defence mechanisms.

THINK ABOUT THIS

Consider these ego defence mechanisms – how can they be applied to your practice? How do you think they will manifest themselves in long-term conditions?

Freud's theory of infantile sexuality and the Oedipus complex

Freud's **theory of infantile sexuality** has its origins in Breuer's earlier discovery that traumatic childhood events have devastating negative effects upon the adult. According to Freud, the newborn infant is essentially an id, driven by the desire for sexual pleasure and demanding total immediate satisfaction. In the early years of life the sexual instinct is satisfied through oral contact, i.e. through the act of sucking and biting the nipple and other objects. Freud termed this the **oral stage** of development. Following the oral phase the locus of sexual gratification shifts to the anus, particularly in the act of defecation; appropriately Freud termed this the **anal stage**.

The penis or the clitoris becomes the focus of the libido during the **phallic stage** during which all children experience the **Oedipus complex**. The Oedipus complex is named after the mythical Greek character Oedipus who unknowingly kills his father and then commits incest with his mother. According to the theory, the complex occurs when the young boy lusts after his mother and so views his father as a sexual rival. Through observation, the young boy realises that girls do not have a penis and comes to the conclusion that it has been cut off by a jealous father (this is termed **castration anxiety**). Anxious to avoid this, boys repress their lustful feelings towards their mother and *identify* with their father by adopting many of their father's attitudes and developing a superego.

While Freud regarded boys' and girls' relationships to the phallus as central to their psychosexual development, the Oedipus complex tends only to refer to the experience of male children. Thus Freud proposed a theoretical counterpart to the Oedipus complex known as the **feminine Oedipus attitude.** (In 1913 Carl Jung proposed the name the **Electra complex** for Freud's concept, deriving from the Greek myth of Electra, who wanted her brother to avenge the death of her father by killing her mother.) The feminine Oedipus attitude or the Electra complex operates in much the same way as the Oedipus complex but in reverse, i.e. girls desire to possess the father and displace the mother. Freud attributes the nature of this psychosexual stage in girls to the notion of **penis envy**. According to the theory, penis envy leads to resentment of the mother, who is believed to have caused the girl's 'castration'. The father figure now becomes the girl's love object and she substitutes her penis envy with the wish to have a child; this ultimately leads to identification with the mother. Following these traumas both sexes enter a **latency period** in which sexual motivations become much less pronounced. This lasts until puberty or what is known as the **genital phase** in which the locus of pleasure or energy release refocuses around the genital area.

According to Freud, the developmental process is essentially a movement through a series of conflicts, the resolution of which is detrimental to adult mental health. Freud believed that many mental illnesses can be traced back to unresolved conflicts which otherwise disrupt the normal pattern of child development. For example, neuroses, paedophilia or homosexuality could be seen as resulting from a failure to resolve the Oedipus/Electra complex, whereas obsessive compulsive disorders concerning cleanliness or hand washing could be seen as failure to resolve conflicts at the anal stage.

THINK ABOUT THIS

Consider how these concepts can be applied to everyday behaviour. Now consider how the Freudian concepts could be applied to mental illness. What does this mean for your practice?

2.4 Evaluation of the psychodynamic approach

Freud is considered as one of the most influential and authoritative thinkers of the 20th century yet many of his ideas have fallen out of favour or have been adapted to incorporate more social rather than sexual influences. A criticism repeatedly made of Freudian and other psychodynamic theories is that they do not easily translate into measurable observations and are therefore un-testable. A related problem is that Freud's (and other psychodynamic) theories are unfalsifiable and therefore lack scientific credibility. During the middle of the 20th century concerns grew about the nature of Freud's data and the validity of the interpretations that he drew from data. For instance, Freud's method of investigation was to focus on the individual (known as an **idiographic approach**), examining particular cases in great detail. Although this has the advantage of providing rich, detailed information, it is hardly justifiable to use such unique observations to formulate general theories about human behaviour. Besides, the case histories that Freud based his theories on were mainly of white middle class women suffering from neurotic disorders; the fact that he relied on such cases to construct a theory of normal development is questionable in itself. Finally, Freud's theories are highly **deterministic** and **reductionist**. They are deterministic to the extent that infant behaviour is determined by innate drives and that adult behaviour is determined by childhood experiences, and overly reductionist because they reduce human behaviour to a basic set of abstract concepts (i.e. the id, ego and superego). Thus too much emphasis is placed on innate biological drives.

Despite much criticism, the psychodynamic approach brings forth several areas that are valuable for the nurse to consider. Firstly, it acknowledges that unconscious desires influence behaviour. Secondly, it recognises that childhood is a critical period of development and that experiences encountered during this time shape future behaviour. Thirdly, it offers an approach for understanding reactions to health problems. An appreciation of psychodynamic concepts, and in particular ego defence mechanisms, will enable the nurse to offer appropriate care and communication. Tailoring communication and care as well as recognising the diverse components which contribute to patient well-being will encourage and facilitate the patient to move forward both physically and psychologically.

Strengths and weaknesses of the psychodynamic approach

Strengths

- Freud's ideas have had a significant impact on psychology.
- Acknowledges that unconscious desires influence behaviour.
- Recognises that childhood is a critical period of development.
- Recognises that childhood experiences are fundamental determinants of adult behaviour.

Weaknesses

- Many psychodynamic concepts cannot be observed or measured (e.g. the Oedipus complex).
- Many psychodynamic concepts are unfalsifiable and lack scientific credibility.
- Theories are post hoc, i.e. based on historical reconstruction.
- Freud's theories were based on a very small, rather unique sample of people and so may lack generalisability.
- Freud's theories are highly reductionist and deterministic.
- Too much emphasis on innate biological drives.

2.5 Behaviourism

Behaviourism was proposed in 1913 by the US psychologist J.B. Watson and monopolised psychology, particularly in the USA, until the early 1960s. Watson, who was influenced by the Nobel Prize-winning work of Russian physiologist Ivan Pavlov (1849–1936) on conditioned reflexes, became increasingly critical of the **introspective approach** which previously dominated psychology. He argued that introspective reports were unreliable and difficult to verify and he made a radical break from traditional introspective psychology. According to Watson:

✳ 'Psychology as the behaviourist views it is a purely objective experimental branch of natural science. Its theoretical goal is the prediction and control of behaviour' (Watson, 1913:158).

According to behaviourists, all behaviour is learnt from the environment (to the near exclusion of innate or inherited factors; this is in keeping with the **tabula rasa view of mind**), can be reduced to simple stimulus response associations and, regardless of its complexity, can be described and explained without reference to internal states (motivation, emotion, etc.) or mental events (i.e. perception, attention, memory, thinking and so on). Thus learning and experience are fundamental to the behaviourist approach.

> **KEY MESSAGE**
>
> **According to behaviourism all behaviour is learnt from the environment.**

Assumptions of the behaviourist approach

- Psychology is the science of behaviour. Psychology is not the science of the mind.
- Only observable behaviour should be studied.
- Behaviour is determined by the environment.
- All behaviour can be reduced to simple stimulus response associations.
- Behaviour can and should be described without making reference to unobservable mental states or internal psychological processes.

2.6 Classical conditioning

Early behaviourist theories suggest that learning and behaviour are the result of conditioning. Conditioning was first reported in the early 1900s by the Russian physiologist Ivan Pavlov. During his experiments Pavlov observed that dogs would often start salivating before their food was presented to them, for example when they saw their food bowl or when they heard the footsteps of the laboratory assistant who was coming to feed them. These observations caused Pavlov to abandon his research on digestion and led to the study of what is now called **classical conditioning**.

Classical conditioning (see Figure 2.2) is a process of learning whereby an initially neutral stimulus comes to elicit a particular response, as the result of being paired repeatedly with an unconditioned stimulus. In the 'language' of classical conditioning, the food in the demonstration above is an **unconditioned stimulus** (UCS) because it naturally evokes an unlearned **reflexive response** (salivation) which is known as the **unconditioned response** (UCR). The sound of the laboratory assistant's footsteps is a **conditioned stimulus**, a previously neutral stimulus that comes to be linked with the food when the two events repeatedly occur close together in time. After satisfactory repetition this too produces a salivation response. When the salivation response is produced by the conditioned stimulus as opposed to the unconditioned stimulus, salivation becomes a **conditioned response** (CR).

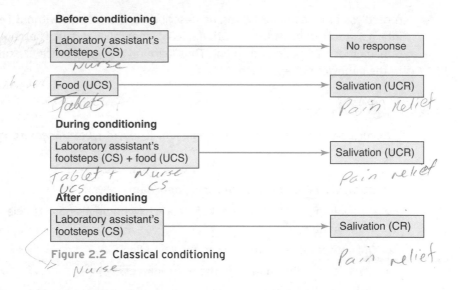

Figure 2.2 Classical conditioning

QUICK CHECK

What are CS and UCS?

There are a large number of successful applications derived from classical conditioning theory. One example that has been widely researched is anticipatory nausea and vomiting (ANV) experienced by patients receiving cancer chemotherapy. Research has shown that prior to treatment approximately 29 per cent of patients experience anticipatory nausea, while anticipatory vomiting occurs in approximately 11 per cent of patients (Morrow *et al.*, 1998). In the 'language' of classical conditioning the first few chemotherapy infusions are the learning trials. The chemotherapy drugs are the UCS that, in some patients, induce post-chemotherapy nausea and vomiting (UCR). During repeated treatments, the hospital or ward, a previously neutral stimulus, is associated with the administration of chemotherapy. Thus the hospital or ward becomes a CS which elicits ANV as a CR in future chemotherapy cycles.

KEY MESSAGE

Classical conditioning can explain physiological reactions to psychological stimuli.

A number of studies provide empirical support for the role of classical conditioning in the aetiology of ANV. For example, Morrow and Rosenthal (1996) report that ANV prior to chemotherapy is uncommon and few patients experience ANV without prior post-chemotherapy nausea. Similarly, Morrow and Dobkin (1988) report that the prevalence of ANV increases with increasing numbers of chemotherapy infusions, while Montgomery and Bovbjerg (1997) found that the severity of ANV increases as patients get closer to the time of their infusion. Although other mechanisms have been proposed, classical conditioning provides the best explanation for the aetiology of ANV in cancer chemotherapy patients (Stockhorst *et al.*, 1998).

THINK ABOUT THIS

How would classical conditioning explain the following:

- a child crying when approached by a nurse;
- an adult with an anxiety reaction to needles;
- anxiety feelings after taking an emetic;
- the use of biofeedback to relax?

An interesting phenomenon in classical conditioning is **stimulus generalisation**. Stimulus generalisation is the tendency of a CR to occur in a weaker form in response to stimuli similar to, but different from, the original CS. For example, it is not uncommon for patients to report ANV when they see the oncology nurse who administers their drugs or when they attend the same hospital for another matter. In one experimental study Bovbjerg *et al.* (1992) found that a new form of drink could induce nausea when paired with several chemotherapy infusions.

THINK ABOUT THIS

How would generalisation be employed within your nursing practice? Consider how this may affect an individual's behaviour in one of the key settings of your practice, whether it be in mental health, physical health or child health, whether in secondary or primary care.

Anti-emetic drugs do not seem to control ANV once it has developed (Morrow *et al.* 1998); so what can nurses do to prevent adverse associations, or if they are inevitable, lessen their effects? According to behaviourists, what can be learned can be unlearned. For example, Pavlov found that when a CS was repeatedly presented in the absence of food, the CR of salivation became weaker and eventually stopped; this is called **extinction**.

THINK ABOUT THIS

How can extinction be used to resolve post-chemotherapy vomiting?

Although prevention is the best strategy (i.e. avoiding post-chemotherapy nausea and vomiting during the initial stages of treatment), a variety of behavioural interventions have been shown to mediate the effects of ANV. For example, **systematic desensitisation** (also called counter-conditioning) appears to have an anti-emetic effect. In this step-by-step approach, patients are taught to replace an anxiety-laden maladaptive response (such as ANV) with an incompatible response (such as muscle relaxation). First, patients are taught progressive muscle relaxation techniques. Next, the patient and the therapist construct what is known as an 'anxiety hierarchy', a list of feared situations relating to the chemotherapy treatment (e.g. driving to the hospital or seeing the oncology nurse). This hierarchy of anxiety-provoking situations is ordered from the least to the most unpleasant. As the patient reaches a state of deep relaxation they are asked to imagine or are confronted by the least threatening situation in the hierarchy. The patient repeatedly imagines or is confronted by this situation until it fails to elicit anxiety, indicating that the counter-conditioning has been successful. This process is repeated while working through all of the situations in the hierarchy.

Several studies have demonstrated the beneficial effects of systematic desensitisation in the treatment of ANV. In one study, 60 patients who developed ANV while undergoing cancer chemotherapy were randomly assigned to receive systematic desensitisation, counselling or no intervention. Researchers found that the frequency and severity of ANV decreased significantly in the group of desensitised patients compared to patients assigned to the other two conditions (Morrow and Morrell, 1982).

THINK ABOUT THIS

How could you use systematic desensitisation in those with a phobia?

Another method based on the principles of classical conditioning (as well as operant conditioning and reinforcement) that has been found to reduce ANV in cancer chemotherapy patients is **biofeedback**. In biofeedback training, patients learn to control a specific physiological response (e.g. blood pressure) by receiving information about moment-to-moment changes in that response. Burish *et al.* (1981) found that when combined with **progressive muscle relaxation training** (PMRT) biofeedback showed promise in reducing anticipatory nausea.

KEY MESSAGE

Classical conditioning can explain some physiological reactions to physical stimuli.

QUICK CHECK

Explain the following terms:

- extinction
- systematic desensitisation
- stimulus generalisation.

2.7 Operant conditioning

Operant conditioning (sometimes called instrumental learning) was first studied by American psychologist Edward Thorndike in the late 1800s. Thorndike's experimental procedure typically involved confining a hungry cat (and, boy, do cats like their food) to a puzzle box from which it could escape and obtain food only by performing a specific behaviour, i.e. operating a latch on the puzzle box door. Each time the cat escaped and ate the food, it was put straight back in and the whole process was repeated. At first the cat struggled to get out, behaving aimlessly until by accident it tripped the latch and managed to escape. However, after repeated trials the cat took less and less time to operate the latch until eventually the cat had learned what to do and could release itself immediately. This led Thorndike to state his 'law of effect'. The **law of effect** states that behaviours (opening the latch) that lead to reward (food) tend to be 'stamped in' (i.e. increase in strength), whereas those that lead to punishment tend to be 'stamped out' (i.e. decrease in strength).

During the 1930s and 1940s, Thorndike's ideas were developed further by the American psychologist B.F. Skinner. Skinner also used a form of puzzle box known as a Skinner box; however, it was modified so that the food could be delivered automatically. In this way the rate of responding could be measured over long periods without having to handle the animal. For example, a rat is placed in a Perspex cage containing a lever or bar. If the lever is pressed a pellet of food will be dispensed. At first the rat presses the lever by accident, but soon learns that there is a link between pressing the lever and obtaining the food. In these procedures, the response being conditioned (i.e. pressing the lever) is called the operant, because it operates on the environment. In turn the food reward is termed a **reinforcer** as it reinforces the likelihood of the behaviour occurring again.

THINK ABOUT THIS

How can you use operant conditioning within your practice?

QUICK CHECK

What is a reinforcer?

2.8 Reinforcement and the token economy system

One of the key concepts derived from Skinner's exploration of operant conditioning was that of **reinforcement**. Wade and Tavris (2003:241) define reinforcement as 'the process by which a stimulus or event strengthens or increases the probability of the response that it follows'. There are two types of reinforcement: positive reinforcement and negative reinforcement. Differentiating between positive and negative reinforcement can be difficult and the necessity of the distinction is often debated. Positive reinforcement occurs when, as the result of behaviour, something pleasurable happens, therefore increasing the likelihood of the behaviour occurring again. So, for example, if every time you behaved in the way I wanted you to, I gave you a doughnut then you would repeat that behaviour. However, there are certain aspects you have to consider when attempting to use these forms of rewards (see Table 2.1).

In contrast, negative reinforcement occurs when, as the result of behaviour, something unpleasant stops; this also increases the likelihood of the behaviour occurring again. For example, an individual who has depression or an anxiety-related disorder may strive to avoid situations that evoke anxiety or unpleasant feelings. The avoidance of anxiety or unpleasant feelings will therefore tend to reinforce the avoidance behaviour.

Operant conditioning describes how behaviour patterns develop through the consequences of that behaviour. An understanding of operant conditioning and the principles of reinforcement will enable the nurse to appreciate what is required in order to enhance or reduce particular patient behaviours. One of the first applications of operant conditioning in the clinical context involved the development of the token economy system. The token economy system is a form of behaviour modification that was often used in psychiatric hospitals to manage the behaviour of individuals who may be aggressive or unpredictable. The system was

Table 2.1 Use of rewards

Aspect	Comment
Timing	The sooner the reward is given after the behaviour the better.
Nature	The reward can be physical (e.g. doughnut, money) or emotional (e.g. smile, praise).
Appropriateness	Ensure that rewards are appropriate – giving an over-weight person a doughnut if they had lost 2 kilos would not be sensible.
Schedules of reinforcement	Continuous reinforcement (i.e. every time you do something you get the reward) leads to quicker learning. Partial reinforcement (i.e. rewards for completing the behaviour are given only part of the time) is learned more slowly but lasts longer.

based on selective positive reinforcement, whereby patients are rewarded with tokens for behaving in appropriate ways; behaviour that is not appropriate is not rewarded. These tokens can later be exchanged for various privileges (e.g. time watching television; cigarettes). Initially tokens are awarded often and in higher amounts, but as individuals learn the appropriate behaviour, opportunities to earn tokens decrease. The amount and frequency of token dispensing is termed a **reinforcement schedule**. Paul and Lentz (1977) carried out a classic study using token economies with long-term hospitalised schizophrenic patients. Researchers found that as a result of the intervention patients developed various social and work-related skills, they were able to take better care of themselves and their symptoms reduced. Remarkably this also coincided with a substantial reduction in the number of drugs being administered to patients. As a result the token economy system has been recommended within mental health psychiatric units (Lin *et al*. 2006).

THINK ABOUT THIS

How would you use reinforcers with the following individuals:

- a person with learning disability being taught cooking skills;
- a person with substance misuse;
- a person with diabetes;
- a person with poor adherence to treatment;
- a colleague who is always late for their shift?

QUICK CHECK

What are the key principles with the use of rewards?

2.9 Evaluation of the behaviourist approach

A large number of successful applications relevant to nursing practice have derived from the behaviourist approach, i.e. behavioural therapy, behaviour modification. In contrast to other psychological approaches, the focus is very much on the patient's behavioural symptoms rather than on the underlying causes of the behaviour itself. This is one of the central criticisms of the behaviourist approach.

Generally speaking the behaviourist approach is grossly oversimplified and mechanistic (machine like). It de-emphasises the influence of knowledge, motivation, subjective experience and emotion, denies the role of innate factors (i.e. the *tabula rasa* view of mind) and excludes the role of cognition. It is a reductionist approach in so far as it reduces complex human behaviour to stimulus response associations and is deterministic to the extent that behaviour is seen as being determined by the environment.

There are ethical problems associated with some forms of treatment based on the behavioural model. For example, most forms of treatment focus solely on behaviour modification and it could be argued that it is dehumanising to neglect patients' internal experiences and feelings. It is also important to reflect on the fact that behaviourist principles are used to control others; this can be seen with the use of token economy systems in psychiatric institutions. Thus therapies derived from the behavioural model can be seen as manipulative. In spite of the criticisms levelled at the behaviourist approach, an understanding of behaviourist theories and associated behaviour modification techniques can help the nurse to understand and discourage maladaptive behaviours.

KEY MESSAGE

Behavioural approaches to some conditions – for example eating disorders – can be viewed as manipulative.

Strengths and weaknesses of the behaviourist approach

Strengths
- Scientific.
- Emphasises objective measurement.
- Large number of successful applications (e.g. therapy).

Weaknesses
- Mechanistic (machine like).
- Reduces complex human behaviour to stimulus response associations.
- Environmental determinism.
- De-emphasises the influence of knowledge, motivation, subjective experience and emotions; denies the role of innate factors and excludes the role of cognition.
- Oversimplified.
- Therapies derived from the behaviourist approach can be seen as manipulative and unethical.

THINK ABOUT THIS

How do the behaviourist and psychodynamic approaches differ?

2.10 Social learning theory

So to recap on the two approaches we have had so far – one has been based on the iceberg of the unconscious and the other on the environment to the exclusion of the 'mind', with the latter being a response to the former (perhaps an over-response?). It is now generally accepted that the behaviourist approach is grossly oversimplified and that it is unlikely that behaviour is solely determined by situational factors. A major alternative to the 'orthodox' learning theories proposed by behaviourism comes from **social learning theory** (SLT).

SLT originated in the USA in the 1940s and 1950s. It is a neo-behaviourist (!!) approach (new behaviourist) because it still emphasises the role of learning as a way of explaining behaviour. However, a central difference between orthodox learning theories and SLT is the introduction of mental states. Although social learning theorists agree that we should only study what is observable, they also believe that there are important cognitive variables that mediate between stimulus and response, without which we cannot adequately explain behaviour. These cognitive (or 'mind') variables cannot be directly observed but can only be inferred from observing actual behaviour. Hence, it is a development of behaviourism rather than an over-reaction to it.

While social learning theorists do not deny the importance of classical and operant conditioning, they do think that these processes provide an inadequate account for the development of novel behaviours.

Assumptions of social learning theory

- All behaviour is learned.
- Classical and operant conditioning cannot adequately account for all human behaviour.
- Cognitive variables mediate between stimulus and response.
- Cognitive variables or mental states cannot be directly observed; only inferred from observing actual behaviour.

QUICK CHECK

What are the key principles of social learning theory?

2.11 Rotter's theory

The first major theory of social learning was put forward by Julian Rotter (1954) who suggested that when we are reinforced for a particular behaviour, this increases our *expectancy* (or belief) that the behaviour will achieve the same outcome again in the future; for example, when we are rewarded for a particular behaviour this increases our expectancy that the behaviour will be rewarded in the future. Thus expectancies are formed on the basis of past experience. It is important to note, however, that expectancy is subjective. There may be no relationship between the individual's assessment of how likely a reinforcement will be and the actual objective probability of it occurring. People can either over- or underestimate this likelihood, and both distortions can be problematic (Mearns, 2008).

> **KEY MESSAGE**
>
> **Expectancies play a key part in reinforcing our behaviour.**

If people have low expectancies, they do not believe their behaviours will be reinforced – so if a person believes their increase in physical activity will not be reinforced by their colleagues then this will impact on the subsequent likelihood of undertaking that behaviour. Consequently they put little effort into their behaviours and are therefore more likely to fail. When they do, it confirms their low expectancies, creating a vicious cycle. When patients have low expectancies, the nurse should endeavour to increase the patient's confidence by helping them to gain insight into the irrationality of their expectancies and/or attempt behaviours they have been avoiding out of fear of failure (Mearns, 2008).

> **THINK ABOUT THIS**
>
> How can you, the nurse, increase an individual's expectancies about:
> - quitting smoking
> - improving their diet
> - being able to take their medication successfully?

Another important concept is the notion of **reinforcement value** – the extent to which we prefer one reinforcer over another when the probability of obtaining each reinforcer is equal. For instance, desirable reinforcers, things we want to happen, or we are attracted to, have a high reinforcement value, whereas undesirable reinforcers, things we wish to avoid, have a low reinforcement value. According to Rotter (1954), an individual may devote a great deal of time and effort to achieve a particular goal because they attach considerable reinforcement value to it. As with expectancy, reinforcement value is subjective, meaning that the same reinforcer can vastly differ in desirability, depending on the individual's life experience (Mearns, 2008). If people set unrealistic or unobtainable goals for themselves, they are likely to experience frequent failure, triggering the development of the vicious cycle described above. In this situation the nurse would help the patient to set realistic, achievable goals – 'it is better to strive step by step, to achieve a series of goals than it is to set one distant, lofty goal for oneself' (Mearns, 2008:4).

KEY MESSAGE

Realistic goals identified as achievable are extremely useful in reaching larger goals.

THINK ABOUT THIS

Using the concept of a series of goals rather than a 'distant, lofty goal' how would you now approach helping a patient:

- quit smoking
- improve their diet
- take their medication successfully?

In the mid-1960s Rotter extended his approach, arguing that some people believe that they have an enormous amount of personal control over the rewards and punishments they receive, while others believe that they have little or no control over what happens to them. Rotter (1966) devised a **locus of control** (LoC) scale to measure these differences. According to Rotter, those who believe that what happens to them depends on their own actions have an **internal LoC**, whereas those who feel that they have little control or that things simply occur by chance or by the actions of powerful agents have an **external LoC**.

2.12 Health locus of control

The concept of LoC was further developed by Wallston and Wallston (1982) who specifically applied it to the area of health; the notion being that those individuals with an internal **health Loc** (HLoC) would be more likely to behave in a health protective manner than those with an external HLoC. Why? Those with an internal HLoC believe that what happens to them depends on their own behaviour and are therefore more likely to take action (e.g. starting an exercise programme or engaging in self-screening behaviours). In contrast, those with an external HLoC believe that what happens to them is beyond their control, down to genetics, fate or God's will and are therefore not convinced that their behaviour will affect their later physical health.

Wallston and Wallston (1982) developed a measure of HLoC. This measure categorised people into one of three types:

- **internal,** if an individual regards their health as controllable by them (e.g. 'I am directly responsible for my health');
- **external,** if an individual believes their health is not controllable by them and in the hands of fate (e.g. 'whether I am well or not is a matter of luck');

- **powerful others**, if an individual regards their heath as under control of powerful others (e.g. 'I can only do what my doctor tells me to do').

If individuals do not value their health, it is thought that they are unlikely to engage in health protective behaviour (even if they feel they have control over their health), because their health is not a high priority.

It should be obvious that people with different types of locus of control will act in a different manner. For example, it could reasonably be expected that those individuals with an internal HLoC or a powerful others HLoC are more likely to behave in a health protective manner compared to those with an external HLoC. However, of course, what action this takes may differ – those with a high internal LoC would be more likely to take their own action, for example starting an exercise programme at the gym. In contrast, somebody with a powerful other HLoC would be more likely to go to a local health clinic and get some diet advice. This type of person would be more likely to seek advice, direction and 'cures' from medical and healthcare practitioners. Those with an external LoC would suggest it was not under their control or was due to other factors such as fate, genetics or God's will.

> **KEY MESSAGE**
>
> **Health locus of control can influence a person's reaction to health messages.**

Norman and Bennett (1995) argue that HLoC is better at predicting health-related behaviour if studied in conjunction with **health value** (i.e. the value people attach to their health). Indeed, Weiss and Larsen (1990) found an increased relationship between internal HLoC and health when health value was taken into account.

In sum, Rotter showed that orthodox learning theories could be extended and improved by adding various cognitive processes (e.g. expectancies and reinforcement value).

> **THINK ABOUT THIS**
>
> How would a person with internal, external or powerful others HLoC react to the following:
>
> - a health promotion message to go for breast screening;
> - a nursing command to stop smoking;
> - some advice to 'lose some weight';
> - an article read in the newspaper?

2.13 Bandura's theory

Rotter's general approach was taken much further by Albert Bandura who tried to reinterpret Freud's concept of identification in terms of conditioning processes. More specifically, he endeavoured to make the concept more 'scientific' by studying it in the laboratory in the form of imitation.

According to this approach, learning can take place both directly through traditional conditioning processes (i.e. classical and operant conditioning) and indirectly through observation. **Observational learning** was first demonstrated by Bandura *et al.* (1961) in the famous Bobo doll experiment. During the experiment children sat and watched a film in which an adult model punched and kicked a large inflated Bobo doll which bounced back every time it was hit. After 10 minutes the children were moved to another room, where there were some toys, together with a Bobo doll. Once in the room they were left to play, during which time they were observed through a one-way mirror. Children who had watched the adult model were violent in their play and imitated some of the behaviours they had observed in the film (see Figure 2.3). In comparison, children who had watched no model or had watched an adult model behave in a non-aggressive manner were non-aggressive in their play activities.

KEY MESSAGE
We learn by observing others.

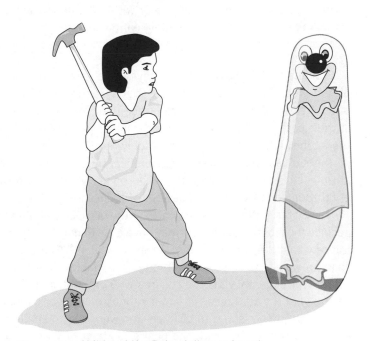

Figure 2.3 **Child and the Bobo doll experiment**

What Bandura's experiment shows is that observational learning can take place without any reinforcement; mere exposure is sufficient for learning to take place. However, whether this learning actually translates into behaviour depends largely upon the consequences of that behaviour. This was demonstrated by Bandura (1965) who investigated **vicarious reinforcement**.

Vicarious reinforcement occurs when another person is observed to be rewarded for a particular action, thus increasing the likelihood that the observer will imitate that action. Bandura (1965) carried out another study in which young children watched a short film of an adult model behaving aggressively toward a Bobo doll. Group one saw a film in which the model kicked and punched a Bobo doll; group two saw the same film, but this time the model was rewarded for their behaviour; and group 3 watched the same film, but the model was punished and warned not to be aggressive in the future. The children were then allowed to play with the Bobo doll. Those children who had seen the model rewarded exhibited the most aggression, whereas those children who had seen the model punished exhibited the least aggression. Bandura wondered whether these group differences in overt behaviour were matched by differences in learning. Accordingly, he rewarded all the children for imitating as much of the model's aggressive behaviour as they could remember. All three groups demonstrated comparable levels of observational learning; however, those who had seen the model rewarded were most likely to apply this learning to their own behaviour.

THINK ABOUT THIS

How would vicarious learning occur within the healthcare setting? Try to think of both physical and mental health examples.

Bandura's SLT explores how individuals learn from observing and imitating others around them. For example, Ost and Hugdahl (1985) report that 12 per cent of adults with a dental phobia can trace their fear back to a vicarious experience in their past. Further research has demonstrated the effects of social learning in the acquisition of dental anxiety in children. Townsend *et al.* (2000) found that mothers of anxious children were significantly more anxious than mothers of non-anxious children, suggesting that children are vicariously developing dental anxiety through observing the behaviour of their parents.

Many interventions have drawn upon the principles of observational learning, especially for those patients who may have a particular fear that becomes a barrier to the care that they are receiving. Melamed *et al.* (1975) provide an example in which children were instructed to sit through a 13-minute film of a four-year-old coping with a typical dental visit. The children who had watched the film of the young boy coping with the visit received lower ratings of anxiety by independent raters and dentists in comparison with children who were shown an unrelated film; they were also more cooperative with the dentist and showed fewer disruptive behaviours.

The principles of observational learning and imitation are equally applicable to student nurses. According to Pearcy and Elliot (2004), students' learning is directly affected by their observations of practitioners and it is only via observing that students are able to develop specific skills. In fact there is evidence to suggest that role **modelling** in the clinical workplace can be one of the most important parts of early nurse education, although it is often underused (Murray and Main, 2005).

THINK ABOUT THIS

How can the nurse use modelling in their practice? Think about it in terms of:

- preparing a patient for surgery;
- working with an adult with learning disabilities to go shopping;
- dealing with an aggressive patient;
- working with children with diabetes requiring daily injections.

KEY MESSAGE

We can model good health behaviour that will result in positive change.

2.14 Self-efficacy

An overarching concept in SLT is **self-efficacy** – an individual's expectation about their capacity to succeed in a particular task. For example, an overweight man who feels that he should do more exercise but has very little confidence that he will be able to do so would be said to have low self-efficacy. In contrast, a woman who is motivated to attend for cervical screening and feels confident that she can do so would be said to have high self-efficacy. Self-efficacy judgements are not concerned with the skills one has but with the judgements of what one can do with the skills one possesses (Bandura, 1977a). Thus the main aim of SLT is to build on self-efficacy, i.e. to enhance the individual's perception of their capacity to succeed.

According to Bandura (1977b), expectations of personal efficacy in any given situation are based on four major sources of information: performance accomplishments, vicarious experience, verbal persuasion and emotional arousal. The impact of this information on efficacy expectations will depend on how it is cognitively appraised.

- **Performance accomplishments** are based on previous experiences of success and/or failure in a given situation. Success raises efficacy expectations, while repeated failures lower them. Once established, enhanced self-efficacy tends to generalise to other situations, although generalisation effects most often occur when activities are similar to those in which self-efficacy was established.

- **Vicarious experience:** many expectations of personal efficacy are derived from vicarious experience. Observing others cope successfully or unsuccessfully in a given situation can generate expectations in observers that they too will succeed or fail if they persist in their efforts.

- **Verbal (social) persuasion:** self-efficacy may increase if an individual is led to believe, through suggestion, that they have the skills required to succeed in a particular situation.

- **Emotional arousal:** high levels of arousal are often associated with stressful and taxing situations, and depending on the circumstances may have informative value concerning personal competency. Because high arousal usually hampers performance, individuals are more likely to expect failure if they are tense and emotionally agitated.

Understanding the concept of self-efficacy is important for the nurse as it can determine (among other things) the initiation of health behaviours (Bandura, 2000), a patient's motivation to follow through with goals that become challenging (Gatchel *et al.* 2007), adherence to medical advice and/or treatment and the successful (or unsuccessful) management of chronic pain (Oliver and Ryan, 2004). Self-efficacy is not just an important determinant of health behaviour but has been shown to be amenable to change; for this reason self-efficacy as a construct has a vital role to play in behaviour modification programmes and patient management.

KEY MESSAGE

Self-efficacy is an important determinant of health behaviour.

QUICK CHECK

What are the four major sources of information that change personal efficacy?

2.15 Evaluation of social learning theory

Although relatively overlooked by other theorists, Bandura's research on observational learning and modelling has been very influential. There is no doubt that observation is important in the acquisition of behaviour; however, Bandura has exaggerated this somewhat. It could also be argued that Bandura's experiments lack ecological validity; there is also the problem of **demand characteristics** as Bandura's experiment almost 'invited' participants to behave in predictable ways. Durkin (1995:406) pointed out:

'Where else in life does a five-year-old find a powerful adult actually showing you how to knock the hell out of a dummy and then giving you the opportunity to try it out yourself?'

On a more general note, SLT has had a considerable impact on nursing and health practice, with major applications in nurse education, patient empowerment, self-management and expert patient programmes. Unlike the other approaches presented in this chapter, SLT clearly illustrates how behavioural, cognitive and environmental factors interact; however, the biological reality underlying cognition and behaviour have been largely ignored, not to mention factors such as emotion and personality. SLT can account for cultural and individual variation in behaviour; it can also explain why we behave in a particular manner in one situation but not in others and this is called **context-dependent learning**. Finally, SLT can be considered a bridge or transition between behaviourist and cognitive theories. We turn to cognitive explanations of human behaviour next.

Strengths and weaknesses of social learning theory

Strengths

- Considerable impact on nursing and health practice.
- Numerous applications.
- Illustrates how behavioural, cognitive and environmental factors interact.
- Can account for cultural and individual variations in behaviour as well as context dependent learning.
- Can be considered a bridge or transition between behaviourist and cognitive approaches.

Weaknesses

- Ignores biological factors underlying cognition and behaviour.
- Does not consider the role of emotion or personality.
- Observers do not always show strong tendencies to imitate the behaviour of a model.
- Bandura's experiments have low ecological validity and high demand characteristics.

THINK ABOUT THIS

Self-efficacy is of key importance in health behaviour and behaviour change. How can you, as a nurse, increase self-efficacy?

2.16 Cognitive psychology

Cognitive psychology first emerged in the late 1950s, a period often referred to as the '**cognitive revolution**', and grew in part out of increasing dissatisfaction with behaviourist explanations. Cognitive psychology is concerned with human thought processes and the ways in which these processes interact with behaviour. There are many facets of cognitive psychology but some of the major areas include memory, learning, intelligence, thinking, and language. Like behaviourism it too rejects introspection as a valid method of investigation and maintains that the only true source of knowledge is that which is obtained through observation and experiment. Yet somewhat incongruous to this is the fact that it explicitly acknowledges the existence of unobservable mental processes. Although there have been many contributors to cognitive psychology, no specific person can be identified as central to its development. What's more, unlike other approaches cognitive psychology does not yet have a unifying theory.

Assumptions of the cognitive approach

- Acknowledges the existence of unobservable mental processes and emphasises their importance in determining and predicting behaviour.
- Accepts empiricist ideas and use of the scientific method.
- Based mainly on laboratory experiments.
- Views the mind as an information processor, i.e. it computes answers to problems in a manner analogous to a computer.

Information processing

Psychologists have often tried to understand human **cognition** by comparing it with something less abstract and better understood. Hence the advent of the modern digital computer provided psychologists with an ideal metaphor for conceptualising how the mind worked and inspired what is now the main **paradigm** within cognitive psychology; the **information processing approach**. According to this approach, the mind is analogous to an information processing system; inputting, storing and retrieving data. This system is used in flexible ways to handle all kinds of cognitive tasks, from reading the newspaper to playing a game of chess. An early version of the information processing approach is shown in Figure 2.4. According to the model, external stimuli are attended to, perceived and then various thought processes are applied to them. Finally a decision is made as to what to do with the stimuli and an appropriate response is produced.

The greatest value of the information processing approach is that it identifies the structures and processes involved in cognition. However, the approach is limited in several ways. Firstly, evidence for the information processing approach is largely based on experiments under controlled, scientific conditions; yet most laboratory experiments are artificial and could be said to lack **ecological validity**. Secondly, although the information processing approach identifies the structures and processes involved in human cognition, it rarely specifies how individuals acquire those processes. You will find the information processing approach discussed further in Chapter 5.

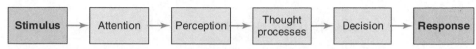

Figure 2.4 Information processing model

Schemas

The concept of **schema** is perhaps one of the most important contributions made by cognitive psychology. A schema is a cognitive structure that contains knowledge about a thing, its attributes and the relations among its attributes (Fiske and Taylor, 1991). It guides individuals and influences how they perceive and interpret events around them and is the basic building block of our cognitive processes.

When we receive information we locate it within a schema (Launder *et al.*, 2005). This saves time and energy through the use of an already established knowledge base. There are many different kinds of schema; for example, schemas about events are called **scripts** and thus guide us when we are performing commonplace activities such as shopping or going to the cinema. **Role schemas** tell us about different roles and how particular groups of people are likely to behave; this would include a schema for a nurse or midwife. Role schemas also include our expectations about social groups and can result in **stereotyping** (see Chapter 4); **self-schemas** embody our self-concept.

QUICK CHECK

What are schemas and scripts?

Schemas are socially determined and derived from our past experiences. They allow us to form expectations and help us to make the world a more predictable place. However, schemas do not necessarily represent reality; thus we can use the concept of schema to explain negative thought patterns or irrational beliefs which are maladaptive to a patient's health and well-being. According to the renowned counsellor and psychotherapist Aaron Beck, some individuals develop self-defeating attitudes as children. Such attitudes often result from past experiences, family relationships or the judgements of others around them. These maladaptive attitudes ultimately develop into schemas against which the child evaluates every experience. The negative schemas of these persons may lie dormant for years. But later in life, upsetting situations such as prolonged stress, illness or hospitalisation can trigger an extended round of negative thinking. Any situation where the patient has negative thoughts or holds beliefs or schemata that are irrational and maladaptive to their health requires the nurse to challenge such beliefs.

KEY MESSAGE

Some people have irrational or illogical beliefs – CBT can help change these.

2.17 Cognitive behavioural therapy

Cognitive behavioural therapy (CBT) combines both cognitive and behavioural principles. The cognitive aspect concentrates on modifying or replacing irrational beliefs or thought processes associated with self-destructive patterns of behaviour, while the behavioural aspect concentrates on modifying or replacing maladaptive behaviours. CBT is most often recommended with disorders and illnesses that encompass anxiety and depression (Curran *et al.* 2006). Most cognitive behavioural experts recommend that CBT is only used by those who have undergone an accredited diploma in CBT (Oldham, 2007); however, nurses will often find that they need to identify triggering factors for particular behaviours and for this purpose the CBT framework is particularly effective.

KEY MESSAGE

CBT is a key treatment modality in mental health practice.

The ABC model

The **ABC model** (Ellis, 1962) is from the **rational emotive** [therapy] component of **cognitive behavioural therapy** and provides a framework that nurses can work within when challenging a patient's negative schemata. Within this framework the nurse will endeavour to change the mental script of the patient so that new ways of thinking will result in behaviour change. The ABC model will encourage the patient to explore the causative factors of their current thinking and to consider the implications of their behaviour. As a result, alternative perspectives that do not result in negative consequences for the patient's health will be sought. Each letter in the ABC model represents a stage, the application of which is as follows:

A. **Activating event** – this could be some action or attitude of an individual or an actual physical event. The patient, with the help of the nurse, could explore triggering factors in this initial stage, which impact upon current behaviour.

B. **Beliefs about the event** – this involves the exploration of irrational beliefs.

C. **Consequence** – this involves exploring the emotional or behavioural consequences of unhealthy negative beliefs or schemata.

D. **Disputing** – the nurse will dispute the cognitive, emotional and behavioural aspects of the patient's current belief system.

Patients can receive many benefits when the ABC model is applied. Firstly, it acts as a catalyst for the patient to reflect on their thinking and to relate their emotional experiences to behavioural reactions. Secondly, it allows the patient to go through a process of self-analysis and self-discovery. Thirdly, it helps the patient understand that people are not disturbed by things or events but by the views they take of them. Fourthly, it helps the patient understand that there are different ways of seeing the same event and thus helps develop alternative ways of thinking. Fifthly, once patients have been educated about the ABC concept, they often report feeling a sense of hope and control (Lam and Gale, 2000). Finally, patients can apply the principles of the ABC model to challenge negative or irrational beliefs outside professional healthcare.

Although the ABC model is most often applied within mental health settings, it may also be helpful to those individuals who:

- hold irrational beliefs,
- distort reality,
- have faulty cognition,
- engage in black and white or all or nothing thinking,
- over-generalise,
- feel they have no control over their lives,
- engage in emotional reasoning,
- feel a sense of hopelessness or **learned helplessness**.

> **THINK ABOUT THIS**
>
> Where could you use the cognitive behavioural approach? How could you use it within your own practice?

Evaluation of the cognitive approach

The cognitive approach has broad appeal and has become very influential in recent years. It focuses on the way that mental or cognitive processes work and the ways in which these processes interact with behaviour. Any explanation that incorporates mental concepts is essentially using a cognitive perspective. What's more, it combines easily with other approaches to produce, for example, social learning theory.

The cognitive approach grew out of discontent with the behaviourist model and its focus on environmental factors; the irony is that cognitive psychology today is rather similar to behaviourism in so far as it excludes certain other internal factors such as motivation and emotion (Eyesenck and Flanagan, 2007). For this reason the cognitive approach has been described as overly reductionist and deterministic. It has also been described as mechanistic because cognitive explanations themselves are based on the 'behaviour' of machines.

Much of the research in cognitive psychology is experimental and conducted in laboratories. Some would argue that laboratory experiments create an artificial environment and that subsequent results have low ecological validity. Nevertheless, there are many successful 'real world' applications of cognitive psychology relevant to nursing and health practice, ranging from suggestions about how to improve communication and information giving, to how theories of perception promote holistic care (see Chapter 5).

Strengths and weaknesses of the cognitive approach

Strengths

- Scientific.
- Large number of successful applications.
- Focuses on processes unique to human beings (i.e. thought).
- Combines easily with approaches, e.g. cognitive behavioural therapy.
- Many empirical studies to support theories.

Weaknesses

- Mechanistic (machine like).
- Lacks human element, i.e. ignores social factors and the role of emotion.
- Research on which cognitive explanations are based is rather artificial.
- Ignores biology (e.g. hormones).

2.18 Humanistic psychology

Humanistic psychology emerged in the 1950s as a reaction to the dominant paradigms in psychology – namely the behaviourist and psychodynamic approaches. Thus it was said to be the 'third force' in psychology by one of its founding members, Abraham Maslow.

The humanistic approach strives to provide a more holistic vision of both psychology and the person. It has roots in **existentialist** thought which holds that human beings have free will and freedom of choice (**personal agency** is the humanistic term for exercising free will). It is further assumed that people are basically good in nature and have an innate need to grow, develop and achieve their full potential; this has been captured by the term **self-actualisation** which will be discussed later. Thus the subjective, conscious experience of the individual is of primary interest; humans are not simply objects of study but must be described and understood in terms of their own subjective views of the world, their perceptions of self and their feelings of self-worth.

KEY MESSAGE

Humanistic psychology is the third force in psychology.

Consequently, humanistic psychology focuses on issues that are uniquely human such as health, hope, love, creativity, individuality and meaning – in a nutshell the personal nature of human experience. The major proponents of this approach are Abraham Maslow and Carl Rogers.

The five main principles that underpin humanistic psychology

- Human beings cannot be reduced to components;
- Human beings have in them a uniquely human context;
- Human consciousness includes an awareness of oneself in the context of other people;
- Human beings have choices and responsibilities;
- Human beings are intentional; they seek meaning, value and creativity.

(James Bugental, 1965)

Maslow's hierarchy of needs and motivations

According to Maslow, the primary cause of psychopathology is the failure to gratify one's fundamental needs. Maslow (1954) outlined these needs within his model (see Figure 2.5), which are presented in order from the most basic needs (deficiency drives) to higher level needs (growth drives). Both drives are leading the person to self-actualisation. Maslow argued that people have to work their way up

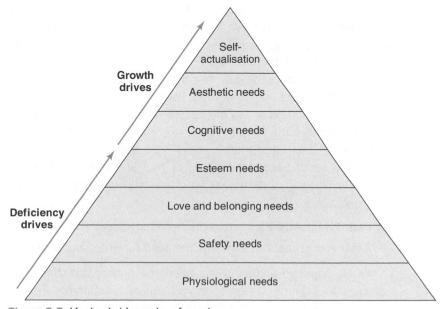

Figure 2.5 Maslow's hierarchy of needs

from the bottom of the hierarchy to the top and that higher order needs cannot be met until lower order needs have been satisfied.

- **Physiological needs:** are the first level of Maslow's hierarchy and encompass the most basic physical needs of the human being (e.g. oxygen, water, protein, vitamins, minerals and so on).

- **Safety needs:** when physiological needs have been satisfied, the need for safety and security comes into play. This level encompasses needs such as protection, stability and freedom from anxiety.

- **Love and belonging needs:** when physiological and safety needs have been met, you begin to feel the need for friends, a partner, children, affectionate relationships in general and even a sense of community. In our day-to-day life these needs manifest themselves in our desire to marry, have a family or be part of a community, church or club. Failure to satisfy these needs can lead to feelings of loneliness and social anxiety.

- **Esteem needs:** next we begin to look for self-esteem. Maslow distinguished between two levels of esteem needs. The lower level is the need for the respect of others, the need for status, recognition, appreciation and dignity. The higher level involves the need for self-respect and includes feelings of confidence, achievement, independence and freedom. Failure to satisfy these needs can result in low self-worth and inferiority complexes.

The levels discussed so far are deficiency drives. If you are lacking at any one level you feel deficient. According to Maslow, all these needs are survival needs; even love and esteem are needed for the maintenance of health. In terms of development, we move through these levels a bit like stages. For example, as newborns our focus is on physiological needs, i.e. feeding or having our nappy changed. Soon we begin to recognise that we need to be safe and secure, after which we crave love and affection; esteem needs soon follow. All of these deficiency drives are encountered within the first few years of life.

Under stressful conditions we can regress to a lower need level. For example, when we are ill we may seek food, liquids, sleep and attention. There is also the possibility of fixation at any of the four deficiency levels. For instance, if you face significant problems during your development, such as the loss of a family member through death or divorce or significant neglect or abuse, you may fixate on a particular set of needs for the rest of your life. This is how Maslow understands neurosis. When all of the deficiency drives have been satisfied, growth drives then come into play:

- **Cognitive needs:** these stem the need for understanding and knowledge.
- **Aesthetic needs:** these include the need for order and beauty.

When cognitive and aesthetic needs have been satisfied the individual progresses to a higher state of psychological functioning. The highest need is referred to as the need for self-actualisation.

● **Self-actualisation:** a number of terms have been used to refer to this need level including growth motivation and being needs (or B-needs). These needs do not involve 'balance' but a continuous desire to fulfil potential; hence the term self-actualisation. Once these needs have been engaged they continue to be felt. This is in contrast to the lower order deficiency needs which surface when unmet. In order to self-actualise, lower order needs must be satisfied: when lower order needs are unmet, you cannot fully devote yourself to fulfilling your potential. It isn't surprising then that only a small percentage of the world's population is truly self-actualising.

QUICK CHECK

List the elements in Maslow's hierarchy.

It is important for the nurse to keep Maslow's hierarchy of needs in mind. This will act as a reminder that many basic needs have to be met before a patient can effectively manage their own state of health. This can also be applied to the nurse and their professional practice – in order for the nurse to work effectively, they should be aware of their own basic needs and ensure they are being met. If not, then the nurse should make this a workable target within their personal development. Many lifestyle behaviours such as smoking or excessive drinking are influenced by multiple internal and external factors. Simply stating that someone has to change will not motivate an individual to do so (Hunt and Pearson, 2001). Instead, motivation itself as outlined in Maslow's hierarchy may need to be addressed before initiating any proposed change.

2.19 Rogers' person-centred approach

By far the most significant practical contribution of any humanistic psychologist is Roger's person-centred therapy (also known as non-directive therapy and client-centred therapy). At the heart of this approach is the basic trust in human beings and in the movement of every person towards constructive fulfilment of their possibilities. Rogers called this a person's 'actualising tendency'. Central to Rogers' theory is the notion of self-concept; the organised, consistent set of perceptions and beliefs about oneself (Rogers, 1959). It consists of the ideas and values that characterise the 'I' and the 'me' and includes perception and valuing of 'what I am' and 'what I can do'. Consequently, the self-concept influences both our perception of the world and perception of oneself. Rogers suggested that if a person's self-concept is close to their ideal self they will experience a high level of self-esteem. On the other hand, if there is very little match the person may experience psychological distress. When a client or patient's actual self and ideal self are distant, it is the role of the therapist or nurse to reverse this situation and help the client become a more fully functioning person.

THINK ABOUT THIS

How can you use the person-centred approach in your practice?

Rogers believed very strongly that people are able to solve their own problems if they are given the opportunity and a supportive environment. He pointed to three core conditions which he described as 'necessary and sufficient' for therapeutic movement to occur. These core conditions are empathy, unconditional positive regard and congruence.

KEY MESSAGE

Empathy, unconditional positive regard and congruence are essential in humanistic psychology.

Empathy

Empathy is the ability to understand what the client is feeling. This refers to the therapist's or nurse's ability to understand sensitively and accurately (not sympathetically) the client's experience and feelings in the here and now.

Many studies have cited empathy as being crucial within any helping relationship. For example, Olsen (1997) examined the relationship between nurse expressed empathy, patient perceived empathy and patient distress. Seventy RNs and 70 patients from medical-surgical acute care units were involved in the study. Each nurse completed two measures of nurse expressed empathy while each patient completed a measure of perceived empathy and distress. Researchers found negative relationships between nurse expressed empathy and patient distress and between patient perceived empathy and patient distress. A moderate positive relationship was found between nurse expressed empathy and patient perceived empathy, demonstrating that empathy is an important aspect of the nurse–patient relationship. Further support comes from Wilkin and Silvester (2007). Forty patients were interviewed and asked to recall a time when a nurse had shown empathy to them, how they did this and any outcomes. The same questions were asked for an occasion when a nurse had not shown empathy. As far as patients were concerned they regarded empathy as important to their recovery process, with one patient stating that engaging in personal conversations 'was the difference between feeing like you were going to die here or go home for Christmas'. Wilkin and Silvester concluded from their study that nurses lacking in empathy cause patients to suffer fear, confusion and depression, lower their confidence in the care provided and subsequently decrease their motivation to comply with treatment.

> **Sympathy and empathy – what is the difference?**
>
> Sympathy has been defined as 'a means to share another's emotions such as sorrow or anguish' (Health and Age, 2006). This differs from empathy, as when expressing sympathy the listener becomes emotionally involved. This can become a barrier to care as becoming emotionally involved may distort clear and measured thinking.

Unconditional positive regard

The next core condition is unconditional positive regard. Unconditional positive regard means that the counsellor (or nurse) must accept the client unconditionally and non-judgementally, irrespective of their illness, lifestyle or previous medical history. It is important that the client is free to explore all thoughts and feelings (good or bad) without danger of rejection or condemnation. Crucially, the client must be free to explore and express without having to meet any particular standards or 'earn' positive regard from the counsellor or nurse.

Unconditional positive regard should be expressed from the outset of the helping relationship, especially when the nurse may not agree with the patient's perspective. In order to display unconditional positive regard, the nurse should not express judgement or expectations towards the patient. In turn the patient will feel accepted and worthy and ready to initiate change.

Congruence

The final condition to initiate change is congruence: also called genuineness. According to Rogers, congruence is the most important attribute in counselling. Genuiness can be defined as 'the basic ability to be aware of inner experiences and to allow the quality of that inner experience to be apparent in relationships' (Rana and Upton, 2009:64). Thus the counsellor or nurse does not present a detached professional façade, but is present and transparent to the client. There is no air of authority and the client does not have to speculate what the counsellor or nurse is 'really' like.

In order for empathy and unconditional positive regard to be successful in initiating change, the patient has to perceive them as genuine feelings. If a patient does not perceive the nurse to be genuine, therapeutic change is less likely to occur. The nurse should be aware that congruence is expressed both verbally and non-verbally; thus self-awareness of one's own behaviour is paramount.

2.20 Evaluation of the humanistic approach

The three core conditions for therapeutic change described by Rogers are key to the understanding of patient-centred care. Likewise, the motivation model provided by Maslow is a useful framework that explores how patients can be motivated to initiate behavioural change.

According to Wilson *et al.* (1996), the humanistic approach isn't a comprehensive theory, but a collection of diverse theories that have similar underlying principles created by people optimistic about human potential. For this reason it has wide appeal to those who seek an alternative to the more mechanistic theories provided by the psychodynamic and behaviourist approaches. Related to this, humanistic psychology has been criticised because its theories are difficult to test empirically. Since humanistic psychology is descriptive rather than explanatory it is subject to what is known as the **nominal fallacy** (Carlson and Buskist, 1997) and so cannot really be called a theory. Humanistic psychology intuitively appeals as positive and optimistic. However, Rogers and Maslow are criticised for having an overly optimistic and simplified view of human nature. Finally, a frequent criticism of the humanistic approach is that delivering the three core conditions proposed by Rogers is what all good counsellors and nurses do anyway. However, this criticism may reflect a misunderstanding of the real challenges of consistently providing the patient with empathy, unconditional positive regard and congruence.

In spite of its shortcoming, the humanistic approach has helped bring the 'person' back into psychology. It recognises that people determine their own behaviour and are not simply slaves to environmental contingencies or to their past (Gross and Kinnison, 2007). However, the greatest contribution of humanistic psychology may lie in its encouragement of humane and ethical treatment of persons, approaching psychology and healthcare as a human science rather than a natural science.

2.21 Conclusion

Contemporary psychology is a complex multidisciplinary subject characterised by a range of different approaches. Given their different assumptions the approaches are sometimes in conflict. Proponents of one approach often criticise the naïve interpretations and treatment efforts of others, yet no approach is complete in itself.

Each approach focuses mainly on one aspect of human functioning and none can explain all aspects of behaviour. Ultimately it is up to you, the nurse, to decide which approach makes best sense to you in the context of the situation you are faced with. According to Raudonis and Acton (1997:138):

'Theory provides nurses with a perspective with which to view client situations, a way to organise the hundreds of data bits encountered in the day-to-day care of clients, and a way to analyse and interpret the information. A theoretical perspective allows the nurse to plan and implement care purposefully and proactively. When nurses practise purposefully and systematically, they are more efficient, have better control over the outcomes of their care, and are better able to communicate with others.'

THINK ABOUT THIS (AGAIN . . .)

On the basis of the material presented here, why do people act in this way:

- yawn
- eat too much
- drink alcohol
- are short tempered
- don't follow your advice
- get depressed
- have phobias about spiders, needles or uniforms?

2.22 Summary

- Psychological approaches to the person attempt to explain why people behave in a certain manner.
- Understanding the person requires an appreciation of a number of psychological perspectives.
- The psychodynamic approach explores how the unconscious mind is responsible for behaviour.
- Freud's psychoanalytic approach suggests behaviour is a result of an interaction between innate drives and early experiences in childhood.
- According to Freud, the mind has three levels: the conscious, pre-conscious and unconscious.
- Freud also assumed that the mind could be divided into three basic sections. the id (innate), ego (reality) and superego (morals).
- The ego protects itself by a number of defence mechanisms.
- Freud's ideas have fallen out of favour or have been adapted to incorporate more social rather than sexual influences.
- A criticism of Freudian and other psychodynamic theories is that they do not translate into measurable observations and are therefore untestable.
- According to behaviourists, all behaviour is learnt from the environment (to the near exclusion of innate or inherited factors).

- Early behaviourist theories suggest that learning and behaviour are the result conditioning (classical or operant).

- The focus of the behavioural approach is on the patient's behavioural symptoms rather than on the underlying causes of the behaviour itself.

- Social learning theorists suggest we should only study what is observable, but believe that there are important cognitive variables that mediate between stimulus and response.

- Expectancies and realistic goals are useful in setting and reaching large goals.

- Health locus of control impacts on an individual's behaviour and response to health messages.

- According to Bandura, we learn by observing others and through vicarious learning.

- Good health behaviour can be modelled by health professionals and will result in positive change.

- An important concept is self-efficacy: an individual's expectations about their capacity to succeed on a particular task.

- Cognitive psychology is concerned with human thought processes and the ways in which these processes interact with behaviour.

- The concepts of schema and scripts are some of the most important contributions made by cognitive psychology.

- Cognitive behavioural therapy is often recommended with disorders and illnesses that encompass anxiety and depression.

- The humanistic approach strives to provide a more holistic vision of both psychology and the person.

- Humanistic psychology focuses on issues that are uniquely human such as health, hope, love, creativity, individuality and meaning – in a nutshell the personal nature of human experience.

- According to humanism, the primary cause of psychopathology is the failure to gratify one's fundamental needs.

- Rogers' person-centred therapy emphasises the basic trust in human beings and the movement of every person towards constructive fulfilment of their possibilities.

YOUR END POINT

Answer the following questions to assess your knowledge and understanding of the schools of thought in psychology:

1. According to Freud the unconscious:

   (a) deals with the here and now

   (b) contains thoughts and feelings from the past that can easily be retrieved from memory

    (c) contains information that the individual is not consciously aware of

    (d) all of the above

    (e) none of the above.

2. The iceberg analogy illustrates:

    (a) the Oedipus complex

    (b) defence mechanisms

    (c) the amount of importance given to the unconscious

    (d) the theory of infantile sexuality

    (e) none of the above.

3. According to Freud's structural model of the mind the id:

    (a) contains innate sexual instincts

    (b) contains innate aggressive instincts

    (c) is located in the unconscious

    (d) all of the above

    (e) none of the above.

4. Classical conditioning is concerned with:

    (a) learning through association

    (b) learning through reinforcement

    (c) vicarious learning

    (d) observational learning

    (e) none of the above.

5. The major proponent of operant conditioning is:

    (a) Watson

    (b) Skinner

    (c) Pavlov

    (d) Bandura

    (e) Upton.

Further reading

Psychological approaches are described and elaborated in most introductory psychology texts.

Armstrong, N. (2008). Role modelling in the clinical workplace. *British Journal of Midwifery*, 16(9), pp. 596–603.

Bandura, A. (1977). Self-efficacy: Toward a unifying theory of behavioural change. *Psychological review*, 84(2), pp. 191–215.

Kreitler, S. (1999). Denial in cancer patients. *Cancer Investigation*, 17, pp. 514–534.

Rana, D. and Upton, D. (2009). *Psychology for Nurses*. Harlow, Essex: Pearson Education.

Stockhorst, U., Klosterhalfen, S. and Steingruber, H.J. (1998). Conditioned nausea and further side-effects in cancer chemotherapy: A review. *Journal of Psychophysiology*, 12 (suppl 1), pp. 14–33.

Thornton, S.P. (2006). Sigmund Freud (1856–1939). *The internet Encyclopaedia of Philosophy*. Available at http://www.iep.utm.edu/f/freud.htm

Watson, J.B. (1913). Psychology as the behaviourist views it. *Psychological review*, 20. Available at http://psychclassics.yorku.ca/Watson/views.htm

Weblinks

http://www.psychexchange.co.uk/index.php
PsycExchange. A resource exchange for psychology teachers with useful video clips including: an interview with Albert Bandura and original footage from his Bobo doll experiments; an interview with B.F. Skinner, showing operant conditioning with pigeons; and an excerpt from a 1960s film about Freud.

http://psychclassics.yorku.ca/index.htm
Classics in the History of Psychology. This site provides a substantial collection of historically significant documents from the scholarly literature of psychology, including original articles written by J.B. Watson, B.F. Skinner, Albert Bandura and Edward Thorndike.

http://www.simplypsychology.pwp.blueyonder.co.uk/
Simply Psychology. This site provides information on the various psychological approaches, including video clips and web links.

http://des.emory.edu/mfp/self-efficacy.html
Information on Self-Efficacy. This site provides a substantial collection of links to self-efficacy and social learning theory.

Chapter 3

Psychology across the lifespan

LEARNING OUTCOMES

At the end of this chapter you will be able to:

- Understand children's development as characterised by Piaget, Vygotsky and Bronfenbrenner

- Appreciate Erikson's staged personality development and its application to nursing and healthcare

- Review how children define and perceive health and illness

- Understand how child development theories can be applied to health and illness

- Understand the definition and extent of 'old age' in the UK

- Appreciate that stereotypes of old people are inaccurate and unhelpful

- Understand the cognitive and social changes that occur in later life

- Explore the nature of death and dying

- Understand the process of grieving.

YOUR STARTING POINT

Answer the following questions to assess your knowledge and understanding of psychology across the lifespan.

1. Piaget proposed that cognitive development proceeded in four distinct stages. What is the correct order?

   (a) Preoperational, concrete operational, formal operational, sensorimotor
   (b) Preoperational, concrete operational, sensorimotor, concrete operational
   (c) Concrete operational, preoperational, formal operational, sensorimotor
   (d) Sensorimotor, preoperational, concrete operational, formal operational
   (e) None of the above.

2. In Piaget's 'conservation of mass' task, children younger than five or six years of age may respond by saying that the lengthened item has increased in mass. What did Piaget conclude from this?

   (a) The child lacks visual acuity.
   (b) The child has an ability to process two aspects of an object at the same time.
   (c) The child cannot 'decentre'.
   (d) The child has the concept of conservation of mass.
   (e) None of the above.

3. What is 'attachment'?

   (a) The behaviour shown when mother and child watch, copy and respond to each other.
   (b) An enduring emotional connection between people that produces a desire for continual contact as well as feelings of distress during separation.
   (c) The ability of a parent to know what a child wants when they cry.
   (d) The emotional connection between mother and father.
   (e) None of the above.

4. Which of the following statements is *FALSE*? In old age:

   (a) Some people find that the marital relationship becomes more rewarding.
   (b) The most long-lasting relationships are usually with siblings.
   (c) Family becomes more important.
   (d) Social networks are no longer important.
   (e) None of the above.

5. What is separation anxiety?

   (a) The child feels fearful when is in the presence of a parent for too long.
   (b) The child feels fearful when the parent tries to leave the child alone.
   (c) The child feels fearful when the parent tries to play when the child is tired.
   (d) The child feels fearful when strangers approach.
   (e) None of the above.

3.1 Introduction

In 2001 there were just under 15 million children in the UK, almost a quarter of the population. Consequently, all nurses will come across children, either during their education, their practice or their personal life. Obviously there may be some nurses that feel that working with children is not for them. However, how children develop and are brought up can have a long-term impact on how individuals behave as adults. Consequently, all nurses – whether they work directly with children or not – need to have an understanding of how children develop and how this has been characterised.

However, development is not just about children as we continue to develop in different ways across our lives. Hence, we need to explore how we develop in childhood, in adolescence, in adulthood and in older age. This chapter will explore development across the lifespan and how psychological theory can be applied in these different stages, and how this theory can be applied to nursing practice.

KEY MESSAGE

Development occurs across the lifespan – from childhood through to old age.

This chapter will start at the beginning – with the newborn and how psychologists, such as Jean Piaget, have attempted to describe how children develop over their early life. The theories of Vygotsky and Erikson will subsequently be explored. Again, these will look at why they are relevant to your education and your clinical practice. Not just if you are working in child health, but also if you are working in adult or mental health or with those who have learning disabilities.

The subsequent sections of the chapter will explore adult development before looking at the older age group, followed by death, dying and the grieving process.

THINK ABOUT THIS

Can you identify any stages of development across the lifespan? Not just from child – adult – older adult, but anything more specialised? Are five-year-olds different from 10-year-olds or 16-year-olds? And so on.

3.2 Piaget's theory of cognitive development

Until the 1930s, children were considered to be small versions of adults. It was assumed that children just behaved differently because they had less knowledge and less experience with the world. Although the flaws with this proposal may now seem rather obvious, this notion characterised much of the thought on child development at the time. Jean Piaget (1896–1980), a Swiss psychologist, was instrumental in developing a theory of cognitive development that fundamentally challenged this viewpoint. Piaget proposed that children do not solely learn on a basis of reward and punishment as suggested by behaviourism (see Chapter 2), rather a child's development occurs through progression through a set of qualitatively different stages. At certain points the child's thinking moves forward and progresses into completely new areas and capabilities. Each of these points can be characterised into different stages:

0–2 years: sensorimotor stage

2–6 years: pre-operational stage

7–12 years: concrete operational stage

12+ years: formal operational stage.

Piaget argued that unless the child had progressed through the stages and was mature enough then they would be incapable – irrespective of how intelligent they are – of understanding things in certain ways. So what are these stages, how were they demonstrated and what do they mean for you as a nurse?

KEY MESSAGE

Children are not simply mini-adults.

QUICK CHECK

What are Piaget's key stages?

The sensori-motor stage

This is the first of Piaget's stages and lasts for the first two years of life. During this time the infant is exploring themselves, the environment and the relationship between these. Infants rely on using their sensory abilities to explore their world, through seeing, touching, listening and sucking (i.e. sensory perceptions and motor activities, hence the sensori-motor stage).

Infants, at this stage, develop important understandings. Firstly, they appreciate that an object can be moved by a hand (they grasp the concept of causality) and develop the notions of displacement and events. Furthermore, children make an important discovery during this stage – the concept of 'object permanence'.

Object permanence is the awareness that an object continues to exist even when it is not in view. For example, infants will lose interest in a toy when it has been covered by a cloth or hidden by a piece of paper (see Figure 3.1). When an infant has developed object permanence (by about eight months of age), when a toy is covered the child will actively search for the object, since they appreciate that the object continues to exist.

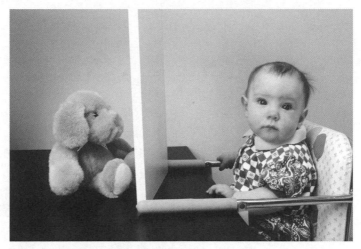

Figure 3.1 **Object permanence**

This is important if we discuss the reactions of the child to their parents. Before object permanence develops, children will usually recognise and respond to their mother (usually by the third day of life) but they will not show signs of distress when left by their mother since she is 'out of sight and out of mind'. However, when object permanence has been developed, if the mother leaves the child then they will show some form of separation anxiety and become upset. This is because the child now appreciates what they have lost – mum!

QUICK CHECK

What do children use to explore their environment during the sensori-motor period?

KEY MESSAGE

During the sensori-motor stage, children become aware of their surroundings and the permanency of them.

The pre-operational stage

Piaget's second stage of cognitive development occurs between the ages of 2–7 years. At this stage children begin to use symbols such as language to represent their earlier sensori-motor abilities. They are now able to use concrete symbolism: they are able to use an object to represent something - a stick as a gun for example. One of the key elements of this stage is that children are still ego-centric - they are unable to take the point of view of others.

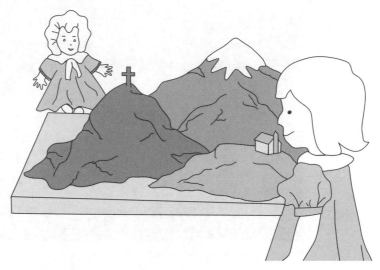

Figure 3.2 **The three mountains task**

In order to test his theory, Piaget developed the three mountains task (Piaget and Inhelder, 1956); see Figure 3.2. In the task, a child is shown a scene of three model mountains which are of different colours. One has snow on top, one a house and the other a red cross. The child is allowed to explore the model and then asked to sit on one side while a doll is placed at a different location. The child is then shown 10 pictures of different views of the model and asked to select which one represents how the doll views it. Piaget and Inhelder concluded that children at the age of four were unable to recognise a perspective different from their own and always selected a picture which matched their own view of the model. Six-year-olds showed some awareness but still often chose the wrong picture. Children of seven and eight years consistently chose the picture that represented the doll's view, supporting Piaget's suggestion that children under the age of seven are egocentric, i.e. they fail to understand that what they see is relative to their own viewpoint.

KEY MESSAGE

During the pre-operational stage, children can use objects to represent things.

QUICK CHECK

What can children do during the pre-operational stage that they cannot at an earlier stage?

THINK ABOUT THIS

How would your interaction with a child with the following differ according to whether they were in the sensori-motor or pre-operational stage:

● a child with a chronic condition,

● a child with a life limiting condition,

● a child requiring surgery,

● a child with an acute illness?

The concrete operational stage

The concrete operational stage is the third stage of Piaget's theory of cognitive development and usually occurs between the ages of 7–11. This stage is characterised by an ability to think logically and organise thoughts in a coherent manner: however, children are not yet able to think in an abstract fashion. At this stage, children are able to comprehend conservation tasks, i.e. the ability to understand that a certain amount of a substance remains the same after its appearance changes.

Piaget developed another experiment to test cognitive development in children, known as a test of conservation. In this task children are shown equal amounts of a liquid poured into two identical containers (see Figure 3.3). The liquid is then transferred into a different shaped container, e.g. a tall, thin container or a short,

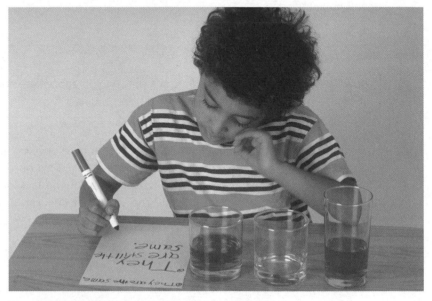

Figure 3.3 Piaget's conservation of volume task

wider one. Children are then asked which container contains the most liquid. Generally, children select the container that appears the fullest even though they have seen that both containers in fact contain the same amount of liquid. Piaget conducted a number of experiments of conservation including: number, mass, weight, volume and quantity. Piaget concluded that children do not develop the ability to conserve prior to the age of five.

KEY MESSAGE

The concrete operational stage is characterised by an ability to think logically and organise thoughts in a coherent manner.

QUICK CHECK

What would the child in the concrete operational stage be unable to comprehend about their nursing care?

The formal operational stage

The fourth and final stage of cognitive development begins at approximately 11 years of age and continues into adulthood. The formal operational stage is characterised by an ability to think in abstract terms, the ability to formulate hypotheses and deduct testable inferences. Piaget suggested that whilst it is possible to achieve such abstract thinking, many people never reach this stage of cognitive development.

THINK ABOUT THIS

How does an understanding of Piaget's theory help appreciate children's understanding of health and illness at different ages?

Despite the impact of Piaget's research on cognitive development, it has not escaped criticism. Apart from the fact that Piaget based his observations on his own children, his work has recently been criticised for the lack of consideration given to contextual factors, specifically the view that children develop within a complex system of relationships and are affected by multiple levels of their environment (Carey, 1985). However, it has had a significant impact on developmental psychology and has been the fundamental underpinning theory of child development for a number of years.

Obviously, the stages of development suggest that children in each of these stages will appreciate health and illness in a different manner. Previous research has linked Piaget's stages of cognitive development to children's beliefs about illness (Bibace and Walsh, 1980) and it is important to develop age appropriate interventions to assist children in their understanding of health, illness and treatment since many children can display unnecessary fear, guilt and anxiety related to health care (Myant and Williams, 2005).

- **Pre-operational stage (2–6 years)**: at this stage children are seen as having limited logic and are highly egocentric. Consequently, children's beliefs about illness are vague with fear and often superstitious. They cannot grasp the finality of death, for example.

- **Concrete operational stage (7–12 years)**: at this stage children begin to understand that ill-health and death have biological causes. Myant and Williams (2005) report that children begin to recognise the risks (in the short term) of their own behaviour and the impact that this may have on their illness/health. In contrast, the long-term outcomes of their behaviour are less understood (Eiser, 1997). However, by the end of this stage children begin to understand that death is final and they begin to understand their own mortality.

Coyne (2006) reported on children's, parents' and nurses' views on the consultation with children in hospital and their participation in care. Results suggested that parents believed that children should be involved in the decision-making process, enhancing and promoting children's self-esteem. Children also indicated the need to be involved in the consultation process in order for them to understand their illness and prepare themselves for procedures. Children's views and opinions were, however, underused. Nurses held conflicting views on the involvement of children in decisions: for some nurses the child's involvement was dependent upon the child's cognitive maturity. Coyne concluded that a health professional's communication is a reflection of their recognition of a child's cognitive abilities rather than their actual competence to understand. In conclusion, Coyne suggested that it is important for nurses to examine their choices about whether to involve children or not in their care and to make explicit decisions with clear criteria for their involvement or not.

KEY MESSAGE

Children should be involved in their care: the extent of their involvement should be determined by the child's cognitive development.

QUICK CHECK

Describe each of Piaget's stages of cognitive development.

3.3 Attachment

Close relationships with the mother (or other primary caregiver) of the child are essential for successful development (and indeed survival in humans) and consequently studies of attachment (and separation) have been reported. The early behavioural approach to the study of attachment viewed the attachment process occurring because the mother provided essential reinforcement for the child in terms of food and comfort. However, a classic animal experiment by Harlow (1959) suggested that this was not an adequate explanation. During this experiment Rhesus monkeys showed a preference for soft physical contact with an inanimate object even if it did not deliver milk. Hence, these studies suggested that children do not just want to be attached to their mothers simply because of the mothers' ability to feed them – they get more out of that relationship in terms of comfort and attachment.

KEY MESSAGE

Infants get more from their interaction with their mothers than simply nourishment.

However, the name most associated with studies of attachment is Bowlby (1969) who noted that babies exhibit a number of behaviours that have a survival value, since the behaviours ensure that the parents (or caregivers) support their basic needs. For example, crying, babbling and smiling signal needs, or clinging and non-nutritional sucking support approach behaviour. Bowlby's theory is based on an interactional model which, as the name suggests, proposes that attachment is dependent on the interaction between the mother and the child rather than being simply dependent on either an infant's or mother's behaviour.

By the ages of 7–12 months, Bowlby noted 'separation anxiety' in babies in as much that they become distressed in the absence of their mother. Consequently, as a result of various studies based on this assumption (notably the seminal studies of the Robinsons during the 1950s), from the 1960s onwards the healthcare system altered to ensure that mothers are encouraged to stay (if possible) during the duration of a child's admission to hospital.

THINK ABOUT THIS

What do Bowlby's studies suggest for the care of children with a chronic illness, particularly those who require considerable time in hospital? How does this alter with the age of the child?

3.4 Ecological systems theory

Another developmental theory needs to be addressed, even though it's not a stage theory, and this is the ecological systems theory of Urie Bronfenbrenner (1917-2005). Bronfenbrenner developed the ecological systems theory to explain how everything in a child and the child's environment affects how a child grows and develops. He labelled different aspects or levels of the environment that influence children's development, including the microsystem, the mesosystem, the exosystem and the macrosystem (see Figure 3.4):

- **the microsystem** – the innermost system that consists of activities in the person's immediate surroundings;
- **the mesosystem** – connections between microsystems, e.g. a child's progress at school depends on parental involvement in school life;
- **the exosystem** – social settings that affect the development of a person, e.g. extended family members, flexible work schedules, etc;
- **the macrosystem** – cultural values, laws and customs of society.

How these groups or organisations interact with the child will have an effect on how the child grows; the more encouraging and nurturing these relationships and places are, the better the child will be able to grow. Furthermore, how

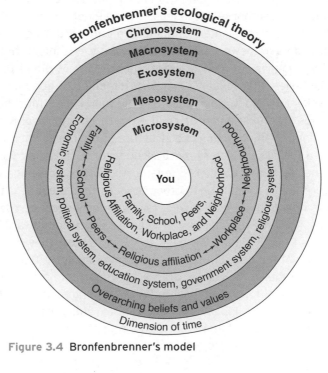

Figure 3.4 Bronfenbrenner's model

a child acts or reacts to these people in the microsystem will affect how they treat the child in return. Each child's special genetic and biologically influenced personality traits, what is known as temperament, end up affecting how others treat them.

THINK ABOUT THIS

How would Bronfenbrenner's model be useful within the healthcare system? What about explaining how best to cope with some of these issues in childhood:

- cleft lip
- diabetes
- anorexia
- substance misuse?

According to Bronfenbrenner's model, the best way to get a valid picture of a child's functioning is to observe that functioning in the context of normal routines and familiar settings. He reminds us that everything we do, believe or understand takes place in a particular social and cultural context and is affected by that context either directly or indirectly. Thus a child's health is affected by environmental factors ranging from family lifestyle choices and cultural norms of behaviour to airborne pathogens. If the aim of modern nursing is to help us seek better ways to maintain and improve our health, then Bronfenbrenner can help provide a framework for such care. Firstly, it is imperative that nurses recognise that health is not understood in a universal way, rather there are cultural and social beliefs that influence our understanding of good health. As parents are the seekers of help for their children then their beliefs must be acknowledged. Sometimes the functioning of children with chronic health conditions may be explained by the function and structure of the family, their cultural beliefs, etc. and so a full clinical history must account for such issues. Furthermore the value of other systems outside of the family should be remembered and the importance of referring a family on to other services should not be dismissed lightly. Another example of the importance of taking an ecological perspective is for the child in hospital – for the majority of children the hospital ward is a new and unaccustomed microsystem. We need to consider how they are going to react and be aware of the needs of the child (and the family) in this setting. Clearly, involving the parents in the child's care will be important here – but the degree of involvement will differ from family to family depending on the child's age, cultural customs and so on. Finally it is important to remember that the family is about more than a child and their parent(s); the role of siblings, grandparents and other family members may also need some consideration

3.5 Vygotsky's sociocultural theory of development

Lev Vygotsky (1896–1934) is another notable theorist of cognitive development. In contrast to Piaget, Vygotsky viewed development as a continuum, with no upper age limit or discrete stages. Vygotsky also emphasised the importance of the social context on development, specifically the influence of social interaction. Vygotsky referred to this concept as the **zone of proximal development** (ZPD) which can be defined as 'the distance between the actual development level as determined by independent problem solving and the level of potential development as determined through problem solving with adult guidance or in collaboration with more capable peers' (Vygotsky, 1978). Essentially, Vygotsky suggested that learning is more likely to occur when there is a 'gap' between what the child can achieve on their own and what they could achieve with the help of someone more skilled.

The concept of the zone of proximal development has been highly influential within the field of education, specifically in the development of peer mentoring programmes. Peer mentoring usually occurs between an older, more able pupil and a pupil with slightly weaker skills. Bruner (1983) developed this further and suggested the concept of **scaffolding**, an interactive process where the more knowledgeable teacher alters the amount of support and guidance required by the child on the basis of the child's responses. In doing so, the child is then able to achieve and develop more.

THINK ABOUT THIS

How can knowledge of Vygotsky's sociocultural theory of development be applied to nursing?

Whilst Piaget's theory tells us comprehensively about the limitations of children's ability to understand concepts related to health and illness, Vygotskian theory provides a framework within which nurses can work to increase children's understanding of what is happening to them in hospital or how to maintain health-related behaviours at home or school. We know from Piagetian theory that there is a stage-related progression in children's use of logic and their interpretation and understanding of health or illness concepts and that this links partly into the child's age. However, that does not mean that a four-year-old should not have the medical procedures they are about to undergo explained to them. Rather it means that the explanation will need to be given in terms and language the child can understand. As Eiser (1989) notes, children will constantly seek to make sense of the world on the basis of their current knowledge and experience. It is therefore essential that children are given accurate information which they *are* capable of grasping fully, in order to diminish the potentially frightening and harmful effects of illness or hospitalisation. Vygotsky reminds us that there is a social aspect to learning and that children do best when taught by more knowledgeable others who scaffold their understanding, and link explanations to experiences and knowledge within the child's own world. This is essential in enabling them to shift from novice to expert in their understanding of their own illness.

3.6 Erikson's theory of personality development

Erik Erikson (1902–94) proposed an alternative theory of child development. In contrast to Piaget and Vygotsky who emphasised cognitive development, Erikson explored personality development. Erikson proposed eight stages in human personality development, beginning in infancy and continuing into late adulthood (see Table 3.1). Each stage is characterised by psychological crises which the individual must resolve in order for a successful adult personality to emerge.

Table 3.1 Erikson's theory of personality development

Stage	Period of development	Description
Trust versus mistrust	Birth–1 year	Warm, responsive area provides infants with a sense of trust and confidence that the world is good. Mistrust occurs when infants have to wait too long to be comforted and they are handled harshly.
Autonomy versus shame and doubt	1–3 years	Using their recently acquired mental and motor skills, children want to be able to decide for themselves. Autonomy is achieved when parents allow a level of independence and do not shame or force the child.
Initiative versus guilt	3–6 years	Through make-believe and creative play, children can develop a sense of ambition and curiosity. Too much control on behalf of the parent is thought to induce excessive guilt.
Industry versus inferiority	6–11 years	At school, children develop the ability to work with others and achieve success. Inferiority develops when negative situations at home or school generate feelings of incompetence.

Table 3.1 Erikson's theory of personality development (*Continued*)

Stage	Period of development	Description
Identity versus role confusion	Adolescence	The adolescent questions their identity and role in society. Exploring values and vocational goals will enable the adolescent to develop a personal identity and positive behaviours.
Intimacy versus isolation	Early adulthood (18-40)	Young adults focus on developing intimate relationships. Failure to achieve basic trust earlier in life may result in an inability to form close relationships as an adult.
Generatively versus stagnation	Middle adulthood (40-65)	In middle adulthood, there is a focus on establishing a successful career and child rearing. Failure to resolve these crises results in an absence of accomplishment.
Ego integrity versus despair	Late adulthood (65+)	During this stage, adults reflect on their life. Those who feel that their life has been worthwhile will experience integrity. Those who feel that their life has been wasted will experience despair and fear death.

According to Erikson, the success of these resolutions and subsequent 'normal' development must be understood in relation to an individual's cultural situation.

THINK ABOUT THIS

How can Erikson's theory be applied to a child growing up with a stigmatising illness such as epilepsy or diabetes?

QUICK CHECK

What are Erikson's stages?

Erikson's theory focuses on the importance of social and emotional develop-ment for children's responses to what is happening to them when they are ill or in hospital. Understanding this model can therefore help the nurse understand and interpret a child's behaviour. For example, a young child who is ill may not fully un-derstand what is happening or why they are in hospital. Providing explanations aimed at their level of understanding using what we know from Vygotsky may help this somewhat. However, children's behaviour may sometimes be at odds with their apparent comprehension and it may be that their social and emotional development holds the key to this. Take for example a 30-month-old child with asthma who is in hospital with a viral infection, suffering from respiratory distress. Oral prednisole has been prescribed as it is known to reduce disease severity and symptom duration for such cases. The nurse is confident that she has been able explain the importance of taking the medicine, yet still the child refuses. Taken at face value, this may appear to be a clear case of a toddler being deliberately difficult. However, according to psychosocial theory this child is in the second of Erikson's stages of personality development and so is striving for autonomy. Refusal to take the proffered medicine may be seen as an attempt to show autonomy. It is important that rather than insisting and getting cross with the child attempts are made to allow the child to take the initiative, in order to mitigate future harmful effects on the child's developing ego.

KEY MESSAGE

Adolescents are not always being truculent but their behaviour is indicative of them striving for autonomy.

3.7 Adolescence – storm and stress

As we mentioned at the outset, rarely do psychologists agree and nowhere is this clearer than in adolescence research. In recent years there has been a dramatic growth in research which has created divergent beliefs and a plethora of psychological theories. Numerous views of the adolescent period have emerged, principally the idea of adolescence as a period of 'storm and stress' (Arnett, 1999; Ayman-Nolley and Taira, 2000). In 1904 Hall proposed that adolescence is essentially a period of storm and stress, a period of psychological turmoil. This, according to Hall, comprised of three specific characteristics: mood disruption, conflict with parents and engagement in risk-taking behaviours. Hall suggested that evolution occurs when organisms pass on their characteristics from one generation to the next, not in the form of genes but in the form of experiences and acquired characteristics (Arnett, 1999). Consequently, the development of the adolescent period, according to Hall, could be associated with some ancient period in evolution that was 'difficult'. This legacy was then passed down from one generation to another and manifested itself as storm and stress in the development of the adolescent period.

Arnett (1999) proposed an alternative view, a modified view of adolescence that incorporates the roles of individual differences and cultural variables. Subsequently, contemporary thought on the issue of storm and stress rejects the notion that it is a universal and inevitable process. Arnett proposes that not all adolescents experience storm and stress, rather adolescence is a period when storm and stress is *more likely* to occur. Consequently, it is important to consider the impact of individual differences and culture upon the development of storm and stress.

Chen and Farruggia (2002), using Bronfenbrenner's model, identify the important role of family, peers and teachers in socio-emotional development during adolescence. Parental warmth, conflict and establishing autonomy are vital factors in emotional development; absence of parental warmth, whether physical or verbal, may result in symptoms of storm and stress. Furthermore, conflict and a desire to establish autonomy during adolescence have also been found as a source of storm and stress (Greenberger *et al.*, 2000). Peer relationships represent a further dimension to the social context of development and have been reported as important for adolescent psychological well-being in different cultures (Greenberger *et al.*, 2000).

THINK ABOUT THIS

What does this mean for your nursing practice when treating an adolescent?

3.8 Putting theories into action

Adolescence is a transitional developmental period between childhood and adulthood. This stage in development can have considerable biological, psychological and social role changes, and probably more of such changes than any other stage of life except infancy (Lerner *et al.*, 1999). Adolescence is a key time for the development of positive health behaviours (e.g. diet and exercise), along with the emergence of health risk behaviours (e.g. smoking, unsafe sex practices and drug use). Thus, the period of adolescence is a good time to try to prevent the bad behaviours from starting rather than attempting to alter them later on.

From the work of Bronfenbrenner we can note that the important others involved with the adolescent include the family, peers, school and work environments – all of which offer the opportunity for preventative interventions. However, some of those listed may be more amenable to interventions than others. For example, peer relationships within the school environment may be one particular focus. Hence, some studies have suggested that improving peer relationships may prove beneficial in improving health behaviours and, for example, recruiting non-smoking adolescents to act as health educators/promoters amongst their smoking peers (Garrison *et al.*, 2003).

When attempting to define target interventions it is important to select appropriate age ranges because of the developmental changes that occur throughout childhood. For example, it could be argued that smoking/obesity, etc. prevention should be directed towards 11- and 12-year-old children and their families for several reasons. Firstly, the body image of children of this age is more malleable as are attitudes towards eating and illness. Hence, although adolescents may struggle with a negative body image and unhealthy eating patterns, the body image of younger children may be more flexible and prevention more likely to succeed (Kater *et al.*, 2000). Secondly, from the age of 11 or 12, children become more autonomous in their health-related self-management behaviours (Pradel *et al.*, 2001). In terms of Piagetian cognitive developmental theory, at the age of 11 or 12 children are entering the 'formal operational' stage (Piaget, 1972) and are developing the skill of abstract thought. Consequently, children at this cognitive stage can begin to imagine the potential consequences (both positive and negative) of a specific health behaviour, which as a result allows them take more control of their health behaviours.

A final concern is that the negative consequences of poor health behaviour may be too far in the future for a pre-formal operational child to imagine (e.g. imagining long-term lung cancer or heart disease as a consequence of smoking). Children may therefore need some concrete and immediate examples for them to consider before they will make their change in behaviour. To deal with this the nurse could ask the child to provide personally relevant examples to ensure they understand the concepts being introduced. It is also important to focus on issues that are most important to children at this age, such as body image (e.g. smoking gives you bad skin and makes you smell when kissing).

3.9 Working with older adults

All nurses, from whichever branch and whatever speciality, need to have an understanding of issues surrounding the care of the older adult. The UK population is ageing, with the 2001 Census estimating that 11 million older people (over pensionable age) were living within the UK. At some stage of your professional career, you will interact with an older adult.

However, the questions that we must try to answer is what is an older adult? How can we define an older adult? What do we mean by 'old'? A simplistic response would be to suggest that it is those over the retirement age (currently 60 years for women and 65 years for men). However, the proportion of people aged over 65 years is considerable and is predicted to nearly double over the next 20 years. Currently, 8.2 per cent of the population are aged 65–74 years, 5.5 per cent aged 75–84 years and 2.0 per cent aged over 85 years. By 2036, the corresponding figures will be 12.5 per cent, 7.9 per cent and 3.7 per cent (Population Trends, 2000). According to Jones (1993), everyone over retirement age is seen as forming a strange homogenous mass, with limited abilities, few needs and few rights: 'What other section of the population that spans more than 30 years in biological times is grouped together in such an illogical manner? . . . As consequence, older people suffer a great deal . . . As for experience and wisdom, these qualities are no longer valued . . . They are devalued by the community, as well as by their owners.'

Thus attempting to define the 'older adult' as anybody aged over the retirement age is compounded with difficulties – a 65-year-old may have completely different needs and expectations from an 84-year-old. Hence, some have suggested that we divide those aged over 65 into three groups: young-old (65–80), old-old (80–90), or very old/oldest old (90+).

KEY MESSAGE

The 'elderly' cannot be considered a homogenous group.

THINK ABOUT THIS

How would you expect a young-old to think and behave in comparison to an old-old, or oldest-old? What specific needs would you envisage for each of the groups?

We also have to consider what people themselves consider as 'old'. Kastenbaum (1979) suggested that there were at least four 'ages of me'.

Kastenbaum's (1979) ages of me questionnaire

- My chronological age is my actual age, dated from the time of birth.
- My biological age refers to the state of my face and body. In other people's eyes, I look as though I am about . . . years of age. In my own eyes, I look like someone of about . . . years of age.
- My subjective age is indicated by how I feel. Deep down inside, I really feel like a person of about . . . years of age.
- My functional age, which is closely related to my social age, refers to the kind of life I lead, what I am able to do, the status I believe I have, whether I work, have dependent children and live in my own home. My thoughts and interests are like those of a person of about . . . years of age, and my position in society is like that of a person of about . . . years of age.

Source: Kastenbaum, R., *Growing Old – Years of Fulfilment*, 1st edn, © 1979. Reprinted by permission of Pearson Education Inc., Upper Saddle River, NJ.

Look at the celebrities in Figure 3.5 and try to guess how old each of them is. Do they act as you would expect somebody of that age to act? How should they act? How do you think a 40, 50, 60, 70, or 80-year-old should act? Is there a stereotypical way you think older people should behave?

Just as it is inappropriate to think of all old people as acting and behaving in a similar way to Tina Turner or Bruce Forsyth, it is also inappropriate to think of the

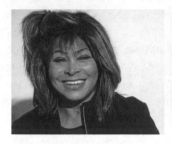
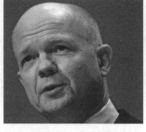
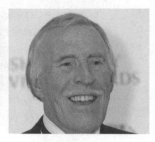

(a) Tina Turner **(b)** William Hague **(c)** Bruce Forsyth

Figure 3.5 **How old are these people?**

older person as doddery, fragile and cognitively impaired. Yet many people continue to hold this view and according to the Ageism Survey carried out by Age Concern (2006), of the 1843 people interviewed about their perceptions of the elderly, it was found that: 'One in three respondents said that the over 70s are viewed as incompetent and incapable' (Age Concern, 2006:3). We all (whether we are nurses or not) have to avoid stereotyping people according to their age. However, this is particularly important for those in the caring professions since it can lead to a self-fulfilling prophecy: 'If you expect older people to be dependent, and consequently treat them as if they are dependent, and encourage them to respond as if they were dependent, eventually they may indeed become more dependent. Low expectations will necessarily lead to under-achievement' (Slater, 1995:17). Similarly, Adler (2000) reports on a number of studies that demonstrate that stereotypes can affect how the elderly think about themselves in ways that can be detrimental to their mental and physical health.

Stereotypes of older people – the elderly – are more deeply entrenched than (mis)conceptions of gender differences. It's therefore not surprising that people are overwhelmingly unenthusiastic about becoming 'old' (Stuart-Hamilton, 1997).

KEY MESSAGE

Stereotypes of the elderly can be widely inaccurate.

WHAT VIEWS DO YOU HOLD OF THE ELDERLY?

Look at each of the following statements (taken from Schaie and Willis, 2002) and say whether they are true or false (the answers are at the bottom of the next page*):

1. Most people over 65 are financially insecure.

2. Rarely does someone over the age of 65 produce a great deal of work of art, science or scholarship.

3. The shock of retirement often results in deteriorating physical and mental health.

4. Old people are not very interested in sex.

5. Old people get rattled more easily.

6. Old people should be active to keep their spirits up.

7. Old dogs can't learn new tricks.

8. In old age, memories of the distant past are clear and vivid, but memories of recent events are fuzzy.

9. Women live longer than men because they don't work as hard.

10. Elderly patients do not respond well to surgery.

11. Most old people become senile sooner or later.

*All are false except 6 and 8.

Odell and Holbrook (2006) suggest that the care that should be provided for older people requires special expertise, because of the following reasons:

- Physiological ageing alters the presentation of disease and effects of medication.
- Incidence of depression, dementia and delirium become increasingly common.
- Pre-existing conditions can make self-care more difficult.
- Social support for successful discharge requires complex organisational skills.

KEY MESSAGE

When interacting with an older adult, do not expect them to act in a stereotypical 'old' manner.

3.10 Cognitive changes in adulthood

There are a number of losses which are associated with **cognitive impairments**. Hall (1988) divides these into four losses. These being:

- intellectual loss – loss of memory, loss of sense of time and loss of expressive and receptive language abilities;
- affective/personality loss – loss of affect, antisocial behaviour and paranoia;
- planning loss – loss of ability to plan activities and functional loss;
- low stress threshold – decreased ability to tolerate stress.

Until relatively recently it was commonly assumed that intellectual capacity peaked in the late teens or early 20s, levelled off, and then began to decline fairly steadily during middle age and more rapidly in old age. However, these cross-sectional studies were methodologically weak and several more recent studies have indicated that at least some people retain their intellect well into middle age and beyond. However, the evidence does seem to suggest that there are some age-related changes in different kinds of intelligence and aspects of memory.

In terms of intelligence, there is some indication that older people's IQ score deteriorates as they get older. Physiological changes can have serious effects on the brain function which, in turn, can impact on intellectual performance. Hence, some have argued that the prime cause of decline in intelligence in elderly people is a slowing of the nervous system processes (Stuart-Hamilton, 2007).

Several aspects of memory appear to decline with age, possibly because we become less effective at processing information (Stuart-Hamilton, 2007). On recall tests the difference is quite pronounced, with the older adult performing more poorly. In contrast, on recognition tests the difference is less apparent and may even disappear altogether. The evidence indicates that for everyday memory, elderly people do have some trouble in recalling events from their youth and early lives (Miller and Morris, 1993).

KEY MESSAGE
Cognitive change is evident with increasing age.

QUICK CHECK
List the cognitive changes associated with ageing.

3.11 Social changes in late adulthood

Cumming and Henry (1961) suggested a social disengagement theory (SDT) to account for an individual's relationship with society, claiming that: 'Many of the relationships between a person and other members of society are severed and those remaining are altered in quality.' This disengagement involves the mutual withdrawal of society from the individual (through compulsory retirement, children leaving home, death of a spouse and so on). As people grow older they become more solitary, retreat into the inner world of their memories and become emotionally disengaged. As far as society is concerned, the individual's withdrawal is part of an inevitable move towards death – the ultimate disengagement.

THINK ABOUT THIS
In light of SDT, are retirement homes a good thing?

Maintaining close relationships with others is often a significant factor in determining whether older people feel a sense of belonging to the social system. This may become important with age, because society withdraws from older adults both behaviourally (e.g. forced retirement) and attitudinally (attributing diminishing powers, abilities and qualities to older people). Hence, there is need for both relatives and friends in a positive older age. Overall, individual adaptation to old age on all levels has been shown to be related to the extent and quality of friendship networks.

THINK ABOUT THIS

How could you increase the friendship network of an elderly patient living alone?

In contrast to the SDT is the activity theory. This suggests that it is the ageist society that withdraws, against the wishes of most people. The withdrawal is not mutual. Since optimal ageing involves staying active and maintaining activities of middle age for as long as possible, and then finding appropriate substitutes during retirement for work and for spouses or friends in the light of their death, it is important for elderly people to maintain a role, to ensure that their role counts and they always have several different roles to play.

KEY MESSAGE

Whatever theory you consider accurate, it is important for the older adult to engage in social activities.

3.12 Dementia

It is estimated that 700,000 people in the UK have dementia. The incidence of dementia increases with age and is thought to double, every five to six years, after the age of 65. In comparison, there are about 18,500 people under the age of 65 with dementia in the UK (Burgess *et al.*, 2006). Dementia is signified with a decline in memory and thinking, present for six months or more, and to a degree sufficient to impair functioning in daily living (World Health Organisation, 1993). There are many types of dementia, including those induced by brain injiuries, tumours, toxins and infections. However, the most common form is Alzheimer's disease which accounts for about half of all cases of dementia. Dementia is a result of a decline in brain function, whatever the cause, and is usually diagnosed on the basis of behavioural reports, psychological assessment and brain scans.

THINK ABOUT THIS

What impact will dementia have an physical and mental well-being? How will this impact on the individual patient and their carer?

KEY MESSAGE

The rates of dementia in the UK are increasing.

One of the main characteristics of dementia is cognitive impairment. Nurses should be aware that dementia care is no longer seen as a collection of deficits, where there is no hope for a patient. Instead, nurses should involve the patient as actively as possible, as well as utilising their strengths and abilities (Burgess *et al.*, 2006). The quality of life can be improved, with adequate communication and specialised individualised care for the patient. By adapting communication so that it is slower and simple will help a patient with dementia feel at ease. However, this does not mean (of course) patronising language, just that it has to be adapted to your patient. Similarly, as we noted above, it is essential that you view dementia appropriately and not in a stereotypical manner, as this influences how the patient feels and the satisfaction they have with the care that they have received.

An elderly person with dementia is more dependent in comparison to an individual without dementia, especially because of psychological, social and behavioural disturbances that accompany the disease. Everyday activities can be disrupted by dementia (Roper *et al.*, 1983) which means that there is a higher need for support even for some of the most basic everyday tasks. An additional concern for many is that the individual with dementia (especially in the early stages of the disease) may become angry and frustrated with both themselves and people around them, because of their dependency. There is an obvious need for the nurse to understand that this may occur and how it can be understood and best dealt with.

Elderly patients are more likely to be treated for their 'present illness', whilst having pre-existing illnesses ignored. For example, Hellzen *et al.* (2003) found that elderly patients who had a diagnosis of long-term schizophrenia as well as suffering from dementia tended only to be treated as a schizophrenic patient alone.

KEY MESSAGE

You must take into account the presenting problem along with the dementia.

The nurse should aim to involve the patient in conversation about themselves, rather than just talking about their present illness. The **person-focused approach** is very much dominant here, with one of the aims being to maintain personhood in the face of failing mental powers (Kitwood, 1997).

Bush (2003) suggests that the focus should be on the person with dementia, not their diseased brain, on the person's emotions and understanding, not memory losses, and on the person within the context of marriage or family and within a wider society and its values. These can be attained with core values that stem from the humanistic approach:

- **Congruence:** What the nurse verbally states should also be displayed via the non-verbal channel or in actions.
- **Unconditional positive regard:** Should be demonstrated by caring for an elderly patient without any conditions or constraints on the relationship.
- **Empathic understanding:** The nurse attempts to understand how the elderly patient, feels, thinks and perceives their symptoms as well as the environment around them.

THINK ABOUT THIS

What does the person-centred approach mean in practice? Discuss with colleagues and come up with some concrete examples.

Communication with a patient with dementia

Feil (1996) suggests that **validation therapy** is the process of communicating with a disorientated older person, by validating and respecting the person's feelings, in whatever context is real to that person at that time, even though it may not connect with the present reality of the hospital setting.

According to Morton's (1997, 1999) **pre-therapy**, there are a number of principles that can be beneficial for nurses who are caring for an elderly patient with impairments. The technique consists of the following reflections:

- situational reflections: used to strengthen contact with the world, and relate to facts, situation, people, environment and events;
- facial reflections: the nurse states the emotion that is apparent in the client's facial expression;
- word-for-word reflections: coherent communication or meaningful sounds are repeated by the nurse in an attempt to support communicative contact;
- body reflections: the nurse mirrors the posture or movements of the patient or reflects them via verbal description.

According to Iliffe and Drennan (2001), concentrating on effective communication with a patient who has dementia is the key to both understanding and resolving behaviour disturbances. Underlying all of these approaches is the emphasis on enhancing the quality of life for the elderly patient by keeping them actively involved. One of these approaches is to focus and utilise the positive resources within the elderly patient and around them. The link between positive attitude and the enhancement of positive health is shown in the media regularly.

KEY MESSAGE

The person with dementia needs to be actively involved in their care.

QUICK CHECK

Give some tips on how best to communicate with a person with dementia.

3.13 Death and dying

The final stage of our development – or ending to be more accurate – is death. Death comes to all of us and it will be a common experience for many nurses. The loss, through death, of loved ones (bereavement) can occur at any stage of life. The psychological and bodily reactions that occur in people who suffer bereavement (whatever form it takes) are called grief. The observable expression of grief is called mourning. We have to recognise that grief can begin before the actual death, and those dying can also grieve for their own death. Nurses have a crucial role to play in helping patients with a terminal illness (along with their friends and families) to come to accept their condition.

KEY MESSAGE

Death comes to all of us. You need to be prepared for your involvement in bereavement and the grieving process.

3.14 Children's understanding of loss

When exploring children's understanding and dealing with loss (infants up until early adolescence), it becomes apparent that there are enormous differences. This can be understood in terms of children's cognitive stage development (as highlighted earlier in this chapter). As a result, the nurse's communication with children who are faced with issues such as loss, grief and death will differ accordingly. Table 3.2 indicates the different grief reactions a child may exhibit depending on their stage of development and highlights the potential input from a nurse or healthcare professional.

Table 3.2 Grief and developmental stages

Age	Understanding of death	Behavioural/ expression of grief	What can the nurse do when caring for a child who is grieving or is terminally ill?
Infants	Do not recognise death. Feelings of loss and separation are part of developing an awareness of death.	Separated from mother – sluggish, quiet and unresponsive to a smile or a coo. Physical changes – weight loss, less active, sleep less.	Awareness by nurse that even though infant does not recognise death they are still affected by the lack of presence of the significant other.
2–6 years	Confuse death with sleep. Begin to experience anxiety by 3.	Ask many questions: How does she eat? Problems in eating, sleeping and bladder and bowel control. Fear of abandonment. Tantrums.	Death here is associated with something that is mystical, magical and peaceful so make sure that your answers reflect these. Giving the chid via non-verbal communication as much security as possible, i.e. comfort, attention, love.
3–6 years	Still confuse death with sleep, i.e. is alive but only in a limited way. Death is temporary, not final. Dead person can come back to life.	Even though saw deceased buried still ask questions. Magical thinking – their thoughts may cause someone to die. Under 5 – trouble eating, sleeping and controlling balder and bowel functions. Afraid of the dark.	Answer acknowledging that concept of death up until about 5 is associated with something magical and peaceful, i.e. daddy is with the angels like you saw him in your dream. From 5 and thereon this begins the process of change to being associated with something that is scary and painful – hence afraid of the dark during the latter phases of this age group.
6–9	Curious about death.	Ask specific questions.	Communication here should take in to account the child's

(Continued)

Table 3.2 Grief and developmental stages (*Continued*)

Age	Understanding of death	Behavioural/ expression of grief	What can the nurse do when caring for a child who is grieving or is terminally ill?
	Death is thought of as a person or spirit (skeleton, ghost, bogeyman). Death is final and frightening. Death happens to others, it won't happen to me.	May have exaggerated fears. May have aggressive behaviours (especially boys). Some concerns about imaginary illnesses. May feel abandoned.	comprehension of death, which has changed from something that is magical and painless to something that is painful and destructive. Even if a parent has protected the child from the subject of death, children will have an understanding from peers, education and the most influential source – the media.
9 years and older	Everyone will die Death is final and cannot be changed. Even I will die.	Heightened emotions, guilt, anger, shame. Increased anxiety over own death. Mood swings. Fear of rejection, not wanting to be different from peers. Changes in eating habits. Sleeping problems. Regressive behaviours (loss of interest in outside activities). Impulsive behaviours. Feel guilty about being alive (especially related to death of a parent, sibling or peer).	Guilt is a predominant feeling when grieving at this stage. Encourage the child to talk as much as possible and work though the guilt. Closing up over a long period of time may result in reference to a counsellor. Peers as a support network are highly beneficial here.

Source: Partly adapted from National Cancer Institute, U.S. National Institutes of Health
http://www.cancer.gov/cancertopics/pdq/supportivecare/bereavement/Patient/allpages/

THINK ABOUT THIS

How would you communicate with a chid that is grieving for themselves, or their mother? Imagine the child is three years old, six years old, nine years old and 12 years old. How does this relate to Piaget's cognitive developmental stages previously outlined?

3.15 Models of grief

According to Archer (1999), a widely held assumption is that grief proceeds through an orderly series of stages or phases with distinct features. Traditional models have one main commonality, the need for grief work, which is described as 'an effortful process that we must go through entailing confrontation of the reality of loss and gradual acceptance of the world without the loved one' (Stroebe, 1998).

Parkes' (1972, 1986) four-stage model describes the phases of bereavement and in turn the grief work that one faces (as displayed in Table 3.3).

The model is very much stage-like; however, the emphasis is on some sort of grief work, with the end result being adjustment to life without the deceased. One way nurses can use this model is to also apply it to terminally ill patients, with the end goal being acceptance of the illness. After all, patients who have been diagnosed with a terminal illness will go through exactly the same grieving process as someone who has lost a loved one and is grieving.

KEY MESSAGE

Grief can be seen as a process of stages, each of which has to be worked through.

Another prime example of a similar stage-like model is that of Kübler-Ross' (1969) five-stage bereavement model, as shown in Table 3.4. This model has provided a framework for caregivers and nurses, working with individuals experiencing personal loss. Kübler-Ross was one of the first researchers to study patients

Table 3.3 Parkes' phases of grief (1972/1986)

Phase	Reactions, emotions in each phase
One	Initial reaction: Shock, numbness or disbelief.
Two	Pangs of grief, searching, anger, guilt, sadness and fear.
Three	Despair
Four	Acceptance/adjustment. Giving a new identity.

and their families from the diagnosis of a terminal illness up until death. It was only after Kübler-Ross' research that more emphasis was given to palliative care and the importance of quality of life even if a patient will die. Also, after the development of this pioneering work death and terminal illness were no longer a taboo subject, and thus it changed nursing/palliative care forever.

QUICK CHECK

List Parkes' and Kübler-Ross' stages of grief.

Table 3.4 Kübler-Ross' model (1969) – the five-stage model

Stage	Example	Explanation
Denial and isolation	'No, not me' or 'It can't be me – you must have the results mixed up.'	During this stage there is constant denial of the new status when a patient or family are told. Denial acts as a buffer system allowing the patient to develop other coping mechanisms. It can also bring isolation and the patient may fear rejection and abandonment in suffering, and feel that nobody understands what the suffering is like.
Anger	'It's not fair – why me?'	This is the stage whereby anger is taken out on practitioners such as nurses (and also doctors, relatives or other healthy people). Typical reactions being, 'because of you (the nurse), I can't go home and pick my children up from school' or 'because of you (the nurse) I have to take time out so you administer pain to me', or 'it's okay for you, you can go home at the end of the day'. Also there is a shift from the first stage from 'no it can't be me, it must be a mistake', to 'oh yes it is me, it was not a mistake'.
Bargaining	'Please God let me . . .'	This is an attempt to postpone death by doing a deal with God/fate/hospital. At this stage, people who are enduring a terminal illness and looking for a cure or 'a bit more time' will pay any price and will usually get manipulated at this stage. It is not uncommon for patients who have never been religious now to turn to religion – almost bargaining

Table 3.4 Kubler-Ross' model (1969) – the five-stage model (*Continued*)

Stage	Example	Explanation
		again – 'if I pray you will grant me another extra couple of days'. The problem is that even when the couple of extra days are granted, these are never enough, the patient wants more.
Depression	'How can I leave all of this behind?'	This time is very much a quiet, dark and reflective period, very similar to someone actually experiencing depression. During this stage, the dying patient does not want reassurance from a nurse, but at the same time does not want to be ignored. During this time family members of the dying patient begin the five-stage model so are very much attempting to be proactive, i.e. in denial that the family member is going to die. They may even become angry at the patient for 'giving up'. The dying patient during this stage would like people around them to be quiet, and this is where nurses can make a difference. All they want is someone to be present who does not question and is not angry. There will be questions the patient will ask and they need to be answered honestly (especially because they don't have to pretend to be strong away from the family). In addition to this, the patient during this stage would also like the nurse to anticipate questions.
Acceptance	'Leave me be, I'm ready to die.'	A stage where the individual is neither depressed nor angry. The individual has worked through feelings of loss and has found some peace. During this stage the patient has let go and is ready to go. Also within this stage, family members are very much angry or questioning why the patient is at peace when they still want to change the status of the patient. The patient, however, has begun the process of letting go during the depression stage and has finished this process of acceptance. They are ready to move on.

THINK ABOUT THIS

What are the problems when applying this model in practice?

3.16 Conclusion

Psychology has attempted to highlight and explain our development from birth through to death. Studies have indicated that cognitive abilities, behaviours and social interactions differ across the lifespan. Knowledge of these differences can assist the nurse in approaching the patient and dealing with any of their concerns.

3.17 Summary

- Development is not just about childhood, it is about changing and developing throughout all of our life.
- Children are not simply small adults.
- Piaget proposed a stage theory – children progress through a set of qualitatively different stages.
- Piaget's stages include the sensorimotor stage (0–2 years), the pre-operational stage (2–6 years), the concrete operational stage (7–12 years) and formal operational stage (12+ years).
- Attachment ensures that children get more from their mothers than simply nourishment.
- John Bowlby noted that babies showed separation anxiety when away from their mothers.
- Bronfenbrenner developed the ecological systems theory to explain how everything in a child and the child's environment affects how a child grows and develops.
- Vygotsky emphasised the importance of the social context on development, specifically the influence of social interaction.
- Erikson proposed eight stages in human personality development, beginning in infancy and continuing into late adulthood.
- The older adult population is ageing, but the 'elderly' cannot be considered a homogenous group.
- Stereotypes of older people (the elderly) are deeply entrenched and can be widely inaccurate.
- There are a number of cognitive losses associated with ageing.

- There are social changes associated with ageing.
- One of the main characteristics of dementia is cognitive impairment.
- The person with dementia needs to be actively involved in their care.
- The loss, through death, of loved ones (bereavement) can occur at any stage of life.
- The psychological and bodily reactions that occur in people who suffer bereavement (whatever form it takes) are called grief.
- Grief can be seen as a process of stages, each of which has to be worked through.

YOUR END POINT

Answer the following questions to assess your knowledge and understanding of psychology across the lifespan.

1. If a child shows secure attachment, what behaviour will they exhibit when a parent returns to them after a brief period of separation?

   (a) Ignore the parent.
   (b) Be indifferent towards the parent.
   (c) Show anger towards the parent.
   (d) Try to reconcile with the parent.
   (e) None of the above.

2. What is adolescent egocentrism?

   (a) The adolescent's belief that friends are more important than family.
   (b) The adolescent's pre-occupation with him or herself.
   (c) The adolescent's desire to start romantic relationships.
   (d) The adolescent's ability to think at the formal operations stage.
   (e) None of the above.

3. Which factor(s) have been identified as critical to maintaining positive mental and physical health in late adulthood?

   (a) having grandchildren
   (b) retirement
   (c) social support
   (d) (a) and (b)
   (e) all of the above.

4. Identify the correct statement from those given below, with respect to peer influence in adolescence:

   (a) Adolescents tend to choose friends who have markedly different interests to their own.

(b) Adolescents tend to choose friends who have similar interests to their own.

(c) Adolescents invariably report that peer pressures have a major influence on their behaviour.

(d) Causation exists between friends' behaviour and adolescents' choices and actions.

(e) None of the above.

5. According to Erikson, what stage of psycho-social development is prominent during adolescence?

(a) trust vs. mistrust

(b) identity vs. identity-diffusion stage of development

(c) autonomy vs. shame and doubt

(d) initiative vs. guilt

(e) none of the above.

Further reading

Baillargeon, R. and DeVos, J. (1991). Object permanence in young infants: Further evidence. *Child Development*, 62, pp. 1227–1246.

Baltes, P.B. and Mayer, K.U. (1999). *The Berlin Ageing Study: Ageing from 70 to 100.* Cambridge, UK: Cambridge University Press.

Brooks, A.M. (1985). *The Grieving Time: A Year's Account of Recovery from Loss.* Garden City, NY: Dial Press.

Dunkle, R.E., Roberts, B. and Haus, M.R. (2001). *The Oldest Old in Everyday Life: Self Perception, Coping with Change, and Stress.* New York: Springer.

Graff, M.J.L., Vernooij-Dassen, M.J.M., Zajec, J., Olde-Rikkert, M.G.M., Hoefnagels, W.H.L. and Dekker, J. (2006). How can occupational therapy improve the daily performance and communication of an older patient with dementia and his primary caregiver? A case study. *Dementia*, 5(4), pp. 503–532.

Kübler-Ross, E. (1969). *On Death and Dying.* New York: Macmillan.

Meins, E. (1997). *Security of Attachment and the Social Development of Cognition.* Hove: Psychology Press.

Schucksmith, J. and Hendry, L.B. (1998). *Health Issues and Adolescents: Growing Up and Speaking Out.* London: Routledge.

Weblinks

http://www.simplypsychology.pwp.blueyonder.co.uk/attachment.html
Attachment. This site contains detailed information on all of the main attachment theories. There is also a video of Harlow's experiment of attachment in rhesus monkeys.

http://www.dementialink.org
Dementia Link. This site provides useful information and support for patients, carers and health professionals.

http://www.compassionatefriends.org
Compassionate Friends. This website offers support for those who have experienced the death of a child.

http://www.piaget.org
Piaget. This site is all about Jean Piaget, the influential developmental psychologist.

http://www.srcd.org
Society for Research in Child Development. This website contains all the latest news and developments in the world of child development, including links to interesting journal articles.

Chapter 4

Social processes

LEARNING OUTCOMES

At the end of this chapter you will be able to:

- Understand the relative contribution of verbal and non-verbal communication in conveying messages

- Appreciate the role of 'attitudes' in influencing our behaviour

- Understand how to modify attitudes

- Persuade people to change their attitudes to healthcare

- Understand how groups affect a person's ability to conform to a particular health regime

- Understand how adherence to advice can be improved

- Realise how the concepts of power and status influence our willingness to conform to healthcare.

YOUR STARTING POINT

Answer the following questions to assess your knowledge and understanding of social processes in nursing.

1. Which of the following is true of Milgram's (1963) study of obedience? The study found that:

   (a) Quite ordinary people taking part in a laboratory experiment were not prepared to administer electric shocks just because an experimenter told them to do so.

   (b) Participants believed that the shocks they administered would not harm anyone.

   (c) Apparently pathological behaviour may not be due to individual pathology but to particular social circumstances.

   (d) (a) and (b).

   (e) None of the above.

2. What were the conclusions drawn about ordinary people based on Milgram's famous study of obedience?

   (a) People will engage in high levels of destructive obedience when faced with strong situational pressures.

   (b) People will engage in low levels of destructive obedience when faced with strong situational pressures.

   (c) People's personality is the strongest determinant of obedient behaviour.

   (d) People will challenge authority figures when they become distressed by their commands.

   (e) (c) and (d).

3. Which one of the following statements about social support is true?

   (a) Social support in a broad social network impacts positively on health and stress.

   (b) Social support in small groups helps one resist pressures to comply with an outside majority or to obey an immoral authority.

   (c) Both (a) and (b).

   (d) Neither (a) nor (b).

   (e) Social support has no impact on health.

4. A change in behaviour or belief as a result of real or imagined group pressure is:

   (a) compliance

   (b) conformity

   (c) acceptance

   (d) reactance

   (e) none of the above.

5. Attribution theory:

(a) was initiated by Leon Festinger

(b) considered how individuals manage to infer the 'causes' underlying the behaviour of others, and even their own behaviour

(c) became influential because it was instantly accessible to the average researcher in North America

(d) was backed up by a large bank of research

(e) none of the above.

4.1 Introduction

Being a nurse means talking and interacting with people. By the laws of probability, just as there must be some donkeys that can tap dance, there will be some nurses that will never talk or interact with people. We can ignore this group of nurses (like we can ignore tap dancing donkeys - see Figure 4.1) and the focus of this chapter will be on all other nurses that do interact with others whether they be your friends, your medical colleagues, your nursing colleagues, other professions or your patients and clients. The aim of this chapter is to explore these social processes and examine how they influence the relationship that individual nurses have with their patients, clients and colleagues and how knowledge of this relationship can assist with your practice. At the start we will look at the importance of **non-verbal communication** (NVC) and how this can be beneficial in any

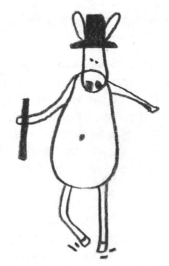

Figure 4.1 A tap dancing donkey

social interaction. This is important, since some studies suggest that almost three-quarters of any message is conveyed by non-verbal communication. This means that the importance of a message is clearly influenced by how we say it rather than what we say.

After looking at non-verbal communication, the chapter will explore the concepts of **attitudes** and **cognitive dissonance**. These concepts are important in healthcare – in whatever form of nursing care you are dealing with. We will also need to explore **persuasion**, and the concepts of **conformity** and **obedience**. How are these related to health and social status? How can these issues and those related issues of **power** and **status** related to the work of the nurse? How are these related to the concept of compliance (or adherence or concordance) to health and how can we manage and increase client empowerment?

Finally, in this chapter we will turn our attention to **stereotyping** and how it can impact on nursing practice.

THINK ABOUT THIS

- List all of the people you interact with in your work.
- What type of relationship do you have with these people?
- What type of techniques do you use to try to alter their behaviour?
- What sort of techniques do they use on *you*?

After all of this, we will need to take a deep breath and have a lie down!

4.2 Non-verbal communication

When we are trying to convey a message to another person, we can do this in a number of ways. The most obvious way is just to say something. 'Have you done your assignment?' can be said and people would understand the meaning of that question, wouldn't they? Well, just with this simple message there will be a number of interpretations depending on the non-verbal messages presented. For example, if we look at each of the 'faces' in Table 4.1 and try to imagine that the simple question had been asked by each 'face' – what would the message be? Would the message be changed?

Non-verbal communication refers to all behaviour which conveys a message distinct from written or verbal language. It includes facial expressions, touch, body movements, postures, arm and hand gestures, and various body movements of the arms and legs. Non-verbal communication is a more subtle communication form than speech and for this reason it can be hard to determine. However,

Table 4.1 **Non-verbal communication**

Face	What would the message be?
Happy	Are you joking?
Serious	Get on and do your assignment!
Angry	Haven't you done it yet?
Sarcastic	You're not going to do your assignment are you?
Worried	You are going to lose marks doing it this late.

non-verbal behaviour is considered important for successful communication. Argyle (1988) suggests that the non-verbal component of communication is five times more influential than the verbal aspect.

KEY MESSAGE

It is not just what you say, but how you say it.

A major goal of effective communication is presenting clear messages, interpreting messages and responding to them in an appropriate way. In any nurse dyad both parties reveal a great deal about themselves through the use of non-verbal communication. For this reason it is essential that all nurses have an understanding of this concept.

Let's look at an extreme example. If you were telling a person they had a life limiting condition, it is unlikely you would do it laughing. Similarly, you would not do it crying your eyes out. Both could be considered inappropriate and may give the wrong impression to the patient. A professional manner would be required in this particular situation. But, of course, the non-verbal communication required in a professional setting may be different from setting to setting and you have to learn how to communicate appropriately, and also understand what the non-verbal communication of the person with whom you are interacting means. Research has found that nursing students show fewer non-verbal communication behaviours than qualified nurses and the authors suggested that student nurses needed to be trained to improve both their own non-verbal communication skills and their understanding of patients' and clients' non-verbal communication (Nishizawa *et al.*, 2006).

THINK ABOUT THIS . . . and try it at home

Have a conversation with a friend about any problems you are experiencing with your nurse training. During the conversation ask your friend to show empathy using verbal and non-verbal communication. Note any non-verbal forms of communication that your friend uses. Now change roles and repeat the task.

Through the use of non-verbal communication we can express either confidence or nervousness which can impact on the confidence of our patients, clients and colleagues. It also provides information about our feelings and intentions (whether someone likes us or not). We can use non-verbal communication to transmit a whole range of different emotions, attitudes, directions, guidance and so on. Indeed any message can be enhanced (or damaged) by non-verbal communication.

So what exactly is it?

Non-verbal communication covers a considerable range of activity from the subtle intonation in a person's voice to the more obvious facial expressions (e.g. grimacing) and hand gestures (e.g. shaking a fist). In Table 4.2, there are a range of non-verbal messages and how they can related to your practice.

QUICK CHECK

List the key areas of non-verbal communication.

Hopefully you can see from the information presented in Table 4.2 how important NCV is in your day-to-day work. Research has explored the use of NVC in nurses. For example, Caris-Verhallen *et al.* (2001) reported that nurses use mainly eye gazes, head nodding and smiling as a means to establish a good relationship with their elderly patients. What is important to note is that the NVC (like any form of communication) should change depending on the situation and the person you are talking to. The way you communicate may be different depending on what message you are giving and to whom you are giving it. Eye gazes and eye contact may be considered the most important and information rich of the non-verbal communication skills used by nurses. But you have to take care: too much eye contact can make a client/patient embarrassed and feel uncomfortable but conversely, a lack of eye contact can be unnerving and worrying.

KEY MESSAGE

Eye contact is important when conveying a message.

Obviously, you also have to learn how to use this skill with your patients – and ensure you take note of how they communicate non-verbally. From this example alone it is clear that elements of non-verbal communication can play an important part in any interaction with either a colleague or a patient. An area in which non-verbal communication plays an essential role is in pain behaviours (for more information see Chapter 7).

Table 4.2 Non-verbal communication

Non-verbal communication	Description	Related to nursing practice
Eye contact	The visual sense is dominant for most people, and therefore especially important in non-verbal communication.	Eye contact is key when giving important information – good or bad news over a diagnosis for example.
Facial expression	Universal facial expressions signify anger, fear, sadness, joy and disgust.	Think about your facial expression when changing a dressing – do you want to show anger or disgust?
Tone of voice	The sound of your voice conveys your moment-to-moment emotional experience.	Tone of voice is of key importance when, for example, trying to reassure somebody with depression.
Posture	Your posture – including the pose, stance and bearing regarding the way you sit, slouch, stand, lean, bend, hold and move your body in space – affects the way people perceive you.	When a client/patient is telling you important information, if you lean forward then you will appear interested.
Touch	Finger pressure, grip and hugs should feel good to you and the other person. What 'feels good' is relative; some prefer strong pressure, others prefer light pressure.	When telling distressing information, touch can be a powerful communicator.
Timing and pace	Your ability to be a good listener and communicate interest and involvement is affected by timing and pace.	When your client is telling you key elements of their mental health you will need to ensure your interventions are appropriately timed.
Sounds that convey understanding	Sounds such as 'ahhh, ummm, ohhh,' uttered with congruent eye and facial gestures, communicate understanding and emotional connection. More than words, these sounds are the language of interest, understanding and compassion.	These **minimal encouragers** can help the patient/client pass on more information.

Another distinct aspect of NVC is touch. Touch is considered a particular type of non-verbal communication and can be particularly beneficial in a therapeutic setting. Five discrete categories of touch were identified by Jones and Yarbrough (1985):

- positive affect (e.g. to show appreciation);
- playful (e.g. to show humour);
- control (e.g. to draw attention);
- ritualistic (e.g. greetings);
- task related (e.g. nurse taking a pulse).

Two of the five categories that are used within nursing practice are positive affect – to communicate reassurance and nurturance – and task-related touch – the use of touch to accomplish tasks such as pulse taking or bathing a patient. Touch has been linked to the phenomenon of caring which in turn fits the concept of nursing practice. Therapeutic touch when used appropriately can be used to convey warmth, empathy and comfort. Reynolds (2002) reported on the usefulness of therapeutic touch when used appropriately in nursing children with cancer.

THINK ABOUT THIS

Where and when would you use each of the categories of touch in your practice?

Again, it is important to know when and with whom to use touch. The use of touch by nurses in adult patients has been shown to have a different effect on males and females (and also whether the nurse was male of female). Whitcher and Fisher (1979) carried out a study where both males and females were touched by a nurse during a pre-operative interaction. Although brief and 'professional' this had a significant effect on post-operative physiological and psychological questionnaire measures. The female patients who had been touched reported less fear and anxiety and had lower blood pressure readings than patients who had not been touched. Unfortunately the reverse was noted in male patients – they were more anxious and had higher blood pressure! Research suggests that these sex differences may reflect more general status differences: people who initiate touch are thought to have higher status than those who receive touch. When the person touching is clearly higher in status than the recipient, it has been demonstrated that men and women react in a positive way to being touched.

KEY MESSAGE

Stop and look – you can learn more from what people do than what they are saying.

However, fear not; although difficult, NVC can be learned and can be developed over the course of your training. For example, Levy-Storms (2008) identified that therapeutic communication techniques including non-verbal communication skills such as eye contact, affective touch and smiling can be taught, and can benefit both nurses and older adult patients' quality of life.

THINK ABOUT THIS

One of your clients with learning difficulties was admitted to hospital for the first time and had very little language capability. The experience of hospital made her very anxious because she did not know what to expect despite some of her carers attempting to reassure her before she was admitted. Her carers recognise her anxiety because of her non-verbal communication – for example, her twitching, her constant eye movement and picking at her clothes. What forms of non-verbal communication could you use to reassure the client?

QUICK CHECK

What is the meaning of the following facial expressions?

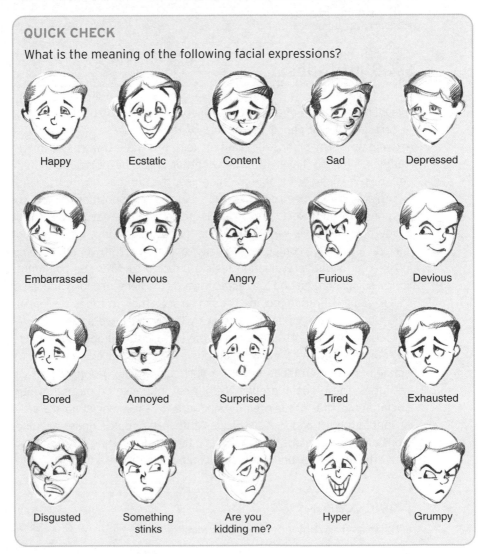

Happy	Ecstatic	Content	Sad	Depressed
Embarrassed	Nervous	Angry	Furious	Devious
Bored	Annoyed	Surprised	Tired	Exhausted
Disgusted	Something stinks	Are you kidding me?	Hyper	Grumpy

4.3 Attitudes

We all have a range of attitudes. Some of these may be benign - attitudes towards a certain make of pencil sharpeners or talented donkeys - others may create an extremely warm or hostile reaction (e.g. attitudes towards religion or sporting teams). All of us have attitudes whether these be our patients, clients or colleagues. We need to be able to recognise these and deal with them appropriately.

An attitude has been described as a learned predisposition to react consistently in response to an object, person or issue in either a favourable (positive) or unfavourable (negative) way. Many argue that attitudes have three components which include a cognitive component (a belief about a person), an affective component (a positive or negative evaluation feeling directed towards the person) and a behavioural component (action is directed towards the person) (Hogg and Vaughan, 2005).

From the definition provided, it can be seen that attitudes are learned - they are not a genetic component that comes with us when we are born - we learn them throughout our life. Attitudes are formed as a result of **observational learning** during our social interactions with various aspects of our environment. Child-rearing, schooling and identification with a particular social group help to construct our attitudes. These **social groups** wield great influence on our behaviour and create social norms that group members adhere to. These social norms are constructed around attitudes and these attitudes influence people's understanding, their reactions and the decisions they make. In a healthcare setting a patient's attitudes may well affect how they understand and follow healthcare advice.

For example, take an individual who has been trying to give up smoking for some time but has been unsuccessful in her attempts. After some time she discusses her attempts with the practice nurse and it becomes apparent that her attitudes are being influenced by family and friends (the so-called 'significant others'). This can indicate that the individual and the family's attitudes can have a key role in influencing behaviour (see Chapter 7). Furthermore, the effectiveness of treatment that is suggested – nicotine replacement therapy (NRT) – to help individuals give up smoking can be influenced by attitudes. For example, if they believe there is a possible risk of addiction to nicotine as a detriment of NRT or that NRT 'was worse than smoking'. Consequently, the attitudes of family, friends and significant others, as well as an individual's own attitudes, can impact on the progress towards quitting smoking.

> **KEY MESSAGE**
> **Attitudes of both the individual and significant others can have a key impact on the success of treatment.**

This shows that attitudes can impact on health from many different directions – the attitudes of the smoker's family have impacted on the support they provide for her and consequently her ability to succeed. Similarly, her own attitude towards NRT is impacting on her use of appropriate interventions and (probably) the success of the intervention. We need to know about people's attitudes because they can affect a person's behaviour. If we know a person's attitude then we should be able to predict their behaviour. Similarly, if we can change their attitude then we may be able to change their behaviour.

Unfortunately, it is not this simple, and some people have reported that there is no relationship between attitudes and behaviour. For example, Gregson and Stacey (1981) found only a small correlation between attitudes and self-reported alcohol consumption. Furthermore, they found there was very little beneficial impact of changing attitudes on changing behaviour.

So, attitudes are as much use as a tap dancing donkey? Why spend time on this concept if it is a complete waste of time? Well, the use of attitudes has been developed further within health psychology to look at so-called 'social cognition models' that can help predict behaviour. For example, it has been demonstrated that a person's beliefs and attitudes about medication can predict treatment adherence (Horne and Weinmann, 1999 cited in Beltran et al. 2007).

These models are explained further in Chapter 5 and this demonstrates the value of attitudes within healthcare practice and how these are essential to alter behaviour and improve health. But what we also have to explore are nurses' attitudes – does the attitude held by a nurse impact on their behaviour? Of course not, nurses are professionals, aren't they? Their attitudes don't affect their actions, do they? Unfortunately, most nurses are humans and despite their professional training and their professional role their individual attitudes will come through. You have to be aware of this – you need to be aware of your own views, your own attitudes and how they affect your practice. Furthermore, you need to be aware of the attitudes of your colleagues and peers – how does this affect their behaviour?

Nurses also have attitudes that may influence how they provide care for patients. Attitudes towards people with mental illness are generally negative in the general population. Nurses may also share similar attitudes. These negative attitudes manifest themselves in the form of bias, distrust, fear, embarrassment, anger, stereotyping and avoidance. Unfortunately these attitudes influence the way a nurse cares for a patient and may also result in many nurses not wanting to work with patients with mental illness.

THINK ABOUT THIS

How you would improve a patient's attitudes towards taking medication for hypertension?

Cognitive dissonance

So attitudes may be positive and we can use these to change the behaviour of our colleagues and our clients. However, what about when attitudes collide? What happens when we have two different views on certain behaviours or towards some belief? According to Festinger (1957), **cognitive dissonance** occurs when a person experiences inconsistencies in their cognitions (thoughts, attitudes and beliefs). Dissonance occurs because a person becomes aware of two or more bits of contradictory information. One clear example of this is in individuals that smoke – they may have one piece of information that suggests smoking is bad for them, and they will have another bit of information (that they get pleasure from smoking). These pieces of information will be inconsistent and hence result in cognitive dissonance.

People prefer consistency in their beliefs, attitudes and behaviours since any inconsistency (dissonance) can cause anxiety and tension. Therefore health-related messages that conflict with an individual's normal behaviour may cause a sense of dissonance (e.g. smoking is harmful to my health but smoking helps me relax).

People seek harmony in their attitudes, beliefs and behaviour and because dissonance is unpleasant psychologically they make every effort to reconcile and resolve their conflicting thoughts. Furthermore, as the dissonance becomes stronger their motivation to resolve it becomes stronger. Festinger (1957) compared dissonance to hunger, arguing that when either occurs humans are motivated to reduce or eliminate it.

THINK ABOUT THIS

Consider the person that smokes who has cognitive dissonance. How will they try to resolve this dissonance? How can this be both positive and negative? How can the nurse use cognitive dissonance to support change in behaviour?

Changing a particular behaviour is often resistant to change since people tend to try to alter one or more of the inconsistent cognitions. Some of the mechanisms that may be used in this endeavour are rationalisation and denial. In the case of the adverse health effects of smoking, people may search for evidence that supports one side of the argument or attack the credibility of the information given. Dissonance can also result in the avoidance of information that could aggravate the dissonance, such as the adverse health effects of smoking. The greater the dissonance, the stronger the attempts to reduce it and one way people try to do this is by avoiding the information in the first place. If the information can be avoided then behaviour change is likely to be very difficult.

THINK ABOUT THIS

Think about the smoker. What has the government done to try to reduce the ability to avoid the message? What can the nurse do to support behaviour change when considering cognitive dissonance?

THINK ABOUT THIS

Think of a time you have experienced cognitive dissonance during your training. How have you tried to resolve this?

QUICK CHECK

What is cognitive dissonance?

4.4 Stereotyping

Related to attitudes are stereotypes. Stereotyping involves classifying people according to generalised characteristics of a particular social group. Stereotypes are often based on attributes such as age, gender, personal appearance, ethnic origin or national or regional characteristics: they are never a representation of what the person is actually like as an individual.

Nurses, like the general public, may be influenced by the stereotyping of individuals. Because of this it is important that an awareness of this concept is understood so that it does not interfere with the development of a good therapeutic relationship between nurse and patient. Usually it is not the positive features of a particular group that are focused upon but the negative ones. Stereotypes and stereotyping are considered by many to be the central component of prejudice and discrimination.

In healthcare, personality types and diagnostic categories are determined through the use of scientifically reliable measures and are usually used to assist in the medical or psychological treatment of patients. However, this type of stereotyping can have negative implications when allowed to take precedence over a patient's personalised medical plan. Nurses bring to the work environment their own biases which may influence the way that patient care is administered.

Rosenthal and Jacobson (1968) demonstrated how damaging stereotyping can be in this classic experiment of self-fulfilling prophecy. The researchers went into a school where they maintained they were evaluating a newly designed IQ test on the students. However, unknown to the teachers, they randomly labelled the students 'clever' or 'ordinary' and made sure the teachers accidentally overheard the names of the students who had done well. The researchers returned at the end of the year and found that students labelled 'clever' had made greater gains than the students labelled 'ordinary'. Observations indicate that students labelled as clever received more attention, encouragement and positive praise from the teacher than the 'ordinary' students. The result became known as the 'Pygmalion effect'. This self-fulfilling prophecy can have implications for patients and the type of care that nurses provide in healthcare settings.

THINK ABOUT THIS

Mandy was a student nurse who had just begun a placement on a surgical ward. John was a patient who had come into hospital for a hip replacement operation. The staff-nurse had told staff that John was diagnosed with schizophrenia and 'may act peculiar' as his hospital notes stated that he suffered from auditory hallucinations. How would you feel if you were in the same scenario as Mandy? Discuss any anxieties and fears you may have about schizophrenia.

It is important that nurses develop a frame of reference, which includes self-awareness and knowledge of their feelings and reactions to certain mental and physical health issues that may have a significant stigma associated with them. Research shows that apart from the development of professional attitudes through education, nurses' direct contact with individuals with mental illness has led to positive attitudes and a reduction in social stigma to people with mental illness. You need to be familiar with the implications of stereotyping and labelling so that these concepts do not interfere with the delivery of personalised care.

4.5 Persuasion, conformity and compliance

So far in this chapter we have discussed people's behaviour and their attitudes. But what about changing, developing or altering people's behaviour and attitudes? Obviously nurses will have to persuade people to do different things. It may range from the mundane – getting your colleagues to make you a cup of tea – to the more important – getting somebody to change a dressing or to help you move something or somebody in an appropriate way. It may be on an individual basis or on a group basis: you may want to persuade your team that you all need to move in a certain direction or change process and policy. You may want to persuade people that what is needed in your unit is a tap dancing donkey (good luck with this one!).

This section will explore the various concepts around persuasion, compliance, authority and power and how we can try to make people do things we want them to do. Obviously, in health and social care we want to try to change people's attitudes and behaviours. We want them to have a negative attitude towards smoking, for example, which is reflected in their behaviour. We want people to have positive attitudes towards certain behaviours – having immunisations, taking exercise and so on. More importantly we want these attitudes to be translated into action.

Persuasion

Persuasion is the process by which an attitude change is brought about. Usually persuasion takes the form of a message that contains arguments for and against a particular attitude.

Persuasive communication was first systematically examined after the Second World War by exploring Hitler's (mis)use of communication and how the Cold War developed and was perceived in the USA (Hovland *et al.*, 1953; McGuire, 1986). Hovland and colleagues (1953) found that for persuasive communication to be effective and to bring about attitude change three variables are important in the act of persuasion, and they developed a model based on their research (see Table 4.3).

Table 4.3 Factors involved in persuasive communication

Factors	Process	Outcome
Source (the sender) • credibility • attractiveness • similarity	Comprehension	Perception change
Message (the signal) • order of arguments • one- vs. two-sided arguments • type of appeal • explicit vs. implicit conclusion	Attention	Opinion change
Audience (the receiver) • persuadability • initial position • intelligence • self-esteem • personality	Acceptance	Action change

QUICK CHECK

What are the key factors involved in communication?

The source of communication (who): the communicator

There are a number of factors associated with the communicator that are important and can have a significant impact on the acceptability of the message to the audience. These variables are highlighted in Table 4.4.

THINK ABOUT THIS

So exploring these factors how can we ensure that our message is received and is acted on? Well, the factors outlined in Table 4.4 are important and relevant to our discussion. How can you, as a nurse, improve your credibility and your attractiveness? What about similarity with your patients? How can this influence your practice?

KEY MESSAGE

Credibility, attractiveness and similarity of the message sender are of key importance when attempting to persuade.

Table 4.4 Communicator factors important in communication

Key factor	Comment
Source credibility	The more credible the source, the more powerful the message and the more likely we are to act on it. Unless, however, the message appears quite bizarre to the receiver – then we tend to question the credibility of the source.
Source attractiveness	Attractive and popular message senders are more likely to have an impact (look at the adverts on TV – most of the actors are attractive).
Similarity	We tend to like people who are similar to us: for example a member of your peer group should be more persuasive than a stranger. However, there are some subtle differences in this. When the query is one of taste or judgement then similar sources are better accepted. However, when the issue concerns a matter of fact then dissimilar sources do better.

The message itself (content)

So far we have spoken about the sender – the person sending the message. We obviously now have to consider the actual message itself. Surely this is the most important component of the trilogy? Obviously the message needs to be conveyed in a manner that will get the point across successfully and effectively. The sender needs the receiver to understand the message and, importantly, be able to act upon it. So we need to explore what characteristics of the message are useful and important, and how we can use these to strengthen our message and our practice.

Several message variables have been found to be important when passing on a message. At the easiest, repetition is both important and necessary. In order for a message to be understood and recalled it helps if the message is repeated often. Indeed, research by Arkes *et al.* (1991) suggests that simple repetition of a message makes it appear truer! Repeating the message appears to influence how the message is stored and accessed in an individual's memory (see Chapter 5) and consequently it is better remembered and, ultimately, acted upon. But surely repetition by itself can become boring and tiresome and make no difference to memory.

One way that many have tried to influence behaviour is through fear. Indeed, fear has been used extensively to try to change health-related behaviours. But of course, such messages can become too fearful and this may have negative consequences. For example, a nurse may visit a school and give a talk on the 'evils of smoking' and try to use fear to get the message over. Similarly, in the 1980s gravestones and the grim reaper were used to try to get the message over about AIDS. More recently, we have pictures of diseased lungs to try to stop smoking behaviour, and pictures of people dying in cars to try to stop people drink-driving. But does this work? Early studies have indicated that there is an inverse-U effect (e.g. Janis, 1967; McGuire, 1969). Keller and Block (1995) argue that using fear at a low level in a message may not be enough to motivate the patient to attend to the message and spell out the harmful consequences of the behaviour. However, a very frightening message may arouse so much anxiety in the patient that they are unable to grasp the content of the message and process the information needed to change the behaviour. But what is a fearful message? This obviously differs depending on the nature of the message and the audience it is being presented to. The fear response may be heightened in children, but certain teenagers may need a more fearful message, especially if they have become desensitised. However, an important message – fear alone does not always result in a change of behaviour.

Sometimes the message can be too powerful to achieve its purpose. A highly emotional message can interfere with the effective processing of the message. It can even result in the person avoiding the message altogether because it causes too much anxiety.

Framing a message in a certain way can influence whether a message is accepted by a patient and leads to a change in attitude and behaviour. When used

125

THINK ABOUT THIS

There are many fear messages on cigarette packets these days, and many other health promotion messages (e.g. about drinking or speeding) try to influence behaviour through fear.

Do these messages work? How do people react to such fear messages?

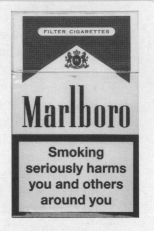

THINK ABOUT THIS

Do fear-arousing messages enhance persuasion? How fearful can a health-related message be to be effective? Think about these audiences: what level of fear could you use?

- getting children to brush their teeth;
- getting teenagers to use condoms with their partners;
- getting older individuals to wear safe slippers when at home;
- getting individuals with schizophrenia to take their medication;
- getting your colleagues to change your rota.

successfully it can be a useful tool in persuasive communication. Rothman and Salovey (1997) carried out a review of how to promote health-related behaviour and found that message framing was an important determinant. They suggest that when the behaviour is regarding detecting an illness, such as breast self-examination, the message is best framed in terms of preventing loss. However, if the behaviour will lead to a positive outcome, such as taking exercise, the message should be framed in terms of gain.

The audience (whom?)

The third element in effective communication is the audience – the receiver of the message. It is important to understand the characteristics of your audience because not everyone responds in the same way to persuasive arguments. We have to be extremely careful when discussing issues with our audience and how the audience has an impact on the message we want to present. Early researchers, Lumsdaine and Janis (1953), suggest that if the patient is against the argument and fairly intelligent you should present both sides of the argument in the message. However, if the patient is already favourably disposed towards the argument and less intelligent it is better to present only one side of the argument. However, a number of problems arise from this observation. What do we mean by intelligence? Does this mean that we should treat less intelligent people unfairly and not give them all aspects of the information? These are a number of points for discussion. However, what you have to remember is that you need to present all information, but that you need to modify how you do this depending on the audience. When you are talking to a colleague your language and tone will differ from when you are talking to a patient. Similarly, how you give this message to your client or patient will differ depending on their background – not just their intelligence but their gender, their age, their social class, their **medical literacy** and so on.

THINK ABOUT THIS

You are giving the following messages to a client with paranoid schizophrenia, a medical consultant and the author of this book. How would your communication change when:

- telling them about a drug regime for heart burn;
- developing a healthy lifestyle;
- telling them about a new system for entering your secure building;
- inviting them to a party?

KEY MESSAGE

You need to change your message depending on the audience.

The channel of communication

The final comment has to be on the channel of communication. The most effective medium for message communication is directly from person to person, whether this be from nurse to patient or from client to consultant. However, written communication needs considerable processing: therefore the use of written information in the form of leaflets can be effective in persuasive communication. However, when writing leaflets and guidance for individuals you have to ensure that you provide material in a suitable format and at an appropriate level for the audience (see Table 4.5 for tips on how to improve written communication).

Table 4.5 How to improve written communication

Desirable feature of the message	Psychological packaging feature(s) likely to help	Physical packaging feature(s) likely to help
That it is noticed	Verbal symbols: 'Warning', 'Danger' Graphic symbol and novelty	Highlighted by use of: colour, border, space, font type and size
That it is legible		Contrast Size of type Avoid text all in capitals Spacing
That it is read	Ensure high readability Use short words Use familiar words Short sentences Avoid negatives Specify vulnerable groups Personalise wording and content Vary wording and content	High legibility
That it is understood	Ensure high readability Explain technical terms Use active rather than passive sentences Be specific in any instructions Use headings wherever possible	High legibility
That it is believed to be true	Cite sources for the message who are likely to be seen as high in: • credibility • expertness • attractiveness	
That it is believed by its target audience	Explicitly mention target groups Deal with counter-propaganda	
That it is remembered if necessary	Ensure high readability Use repetition Use specific/concrete statements Use explicit categorisation Use primacy effect	Highlighting parts of the message which need to be remembered

Conformity, obedience and compliance

We now move on to changing people's behaviour through conformity, obedience and compliance. These three elements are all linked and provide an important foundation for understanding the relationship between the nurse and client/patient and that with colleagues.

Conformity is the first element to discuss and can be defined as a social influence which involves a person's attitude and behaviour yielding to group pressure from a particular social group. Conformity affects our attitudes and behaviours and can affect a patient's adherence to healthcare advice.

The most famous study on conformity was undertaken in the 1950s by Asch (1952). He aimed to investigate how people are affected by group pressure to conform to a particular behaviour. Participants were told that they were taking part in a task that involved visual judgement. During the task they were shown a line on a piece of card. They were then asked to match the line with three lines on a different card. Unknown to the participant they were put in a room with a number of confederates of the researcher who were asked to select the incorrect line. In Figure 4.2, the confederates were asked to say that line A in the comparison list was exactly the same length as the standard, despite the fact that the obvious correct answer is line B.

During the task 50 per cent of the participants conformed to the majority, selecting the same incorrect line as the confederates. Only 25 per cent remained independent of the group pressure and selected the correct line.

> **THINK ABOUT THIS**
>
> The Asch study was conducted in the 1950s. Do you think the same thing would happen these days? Do you think nurses conform? The last time you were on a ward, was there an occasion where you conformed because you thought you had to?

Many studies have explored the Asch effect and some have suggested that it was a 'child of its time'. However, there is considerable research evidence that confirms it is both a consistent effect and one that can be observed across cultures and times (e.g. Takano and Sogon, 2008).

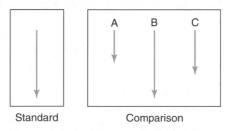

Figure 4.2 Asch's presentation of lines

But what relevance has this for nursing? Do you think it has an impact on you? Well, if we think of the example provided in the following box – a case from professional practice – what would you do in this situation?

Professional practice issues

In professional practice, a third year student nurse (Colin) was on a placement on a geriatric ward. During the placement he observed that patients were not being turned on a regular basis as recommended in his training and as he had observed on other wards. When he pointed this out to a more experienced nurse she became agitated and informed him that this was a very busy ward and they had their own way of doing things. He took this to a team meeting and all of his colleagues also reported that this was the case. The student nurse was in a minority of one and hence had a dilemma: would he conform to the majority and compromise the quality of patient care or would he seek advice from his practice facilitator and upset the rest of the team?

For student nurses the need to conform can be strong. Many lack confidence because of their inexperience and feel discourteous when pointing out concerns to more experienced and qualified members of the team. Sometimes roles and available knowledge are ambiguous. The need to fit in and gain approval can sometimes cloud a nurse's judgement. However, the patients' needs must always take priority over the group norm and it is important that nurses are aware of this.

QUICK CHECK

What are conformity and obedience?

Compliance

Compliance is generally viewed as the degree to which medical advice is followed in order to reach a therapeutic goal (Kelly, 1995). At this stage, we need to consider the term compliance and whether this term is appropriate. Often, the terms 'compliance' and 'adherence' are used interchangeably. The term **compliance** was frequently used during the early stages of research, which investigated the patient following (or not) their practitioner's instructions. Haynes *et al.* (1979) defined compliance as:

> 'The extent to which the patient's behaviour, (in terms of taking medication, following diets or other lifestyle changes) coincides with medical or health advice.'

The term compliance implies that the patient will follow the nurse's orders without any questions, is always in a less informed position and that a failure to comply is the fault of the patient (Waitzkin, 1989; Donovan and Blake, 1992). This term has been heavily criticised in nursing literature for its paternalistic view of the health professional-patient relationship, in which the patient is perceived to be passive and expected to obey the clinician's orders (Snelgrove, 2006). Many nurses feel uneasy about the label, as it directs blame largely towards the patient (Russell *et al.*, 2003). Consequently, the term 'adherence' was employed, but again this was criticised and more recently the term concordance (i.e. alignment of the patient's and the nurse's views - a partnership) is preferred. In this chapter we will use these three terms interchangeably (although we prefer the term concordance) depending on the nature of the research being reported.

THINK ABOUT THIS

What sort of factors do you think might cause non-compliance with the medical advice given for the treatment of hypertension?

Recent research has shown that when patients feel they are actively involved in their treatment, adherence levels to treatment increase. Therefore the term concordance has been introduced by some in healthcare to represent a shared understanding between healthcare professionals and patients about their care, treatment and management (Ogden, 2007).

KEY MESSAGE

People do not always follow medical and nursing advice.

Compliance is considered to be a determinant of patient well-being. However, as already mentioned, many patients do not comply with the healthcare advice given. Therefore we have to pose the question: what are the factors that influence compliance to medical advice? The principal reasons that have been identified for poor compliance include adverse effects, forgetfulness, changing priorities or schedules and confusion about dosing regimens. The relationship between the patient and the healthcare provider has also been considered.

Phillip Ley (1981, 1989) developed the **cognitive hypothesis model of compliance.** According to this model, patient compliance can be predicted by:

- patient satisfaction with the process of the consultation;
- understanding of the information provided during the consultation; and
- the recall of this information.

THINK ABOUT THIS

What aspect of the nurse–patient consultation would result in patient satisfaction?

A study investigating the role of some of the factors highlighted by Kreuter *et al.* (2000) showed that increased patient education can lead to higher rates of 'conformity' and better health outcomes. Patients' ability to recall the information that the nurse has conveyed to them is influenced by a multitude of factors such as anxiety, the primacy effect (the tendency for the information that is presented first to be remembered), medical knowledge, intellectual level and the importance of the statement. This will be explored in further detail in Chapter 5.

QUICK CHECK

- Describe the three variables that Hovland and associates (1953) suggest are important in the communication of persuasion.
- Explain how the concept of conformity can affect a patient's willingness to reduce the amount of alcohol they consume.
- In a group, discuss some of the factors that may influence an adolescent patient's willingness to continue taking insulin for juvenile rheumatoid arthritis.

4.6 Power and status

As highlighted above, the concept of compliance or adherence can be influenced by the principles of persuasion as discussed above. Furthermore, it can also be influenced by how much power a person is perceived to have. Power is the capacity of one person to influence another individual to do what the influencer wants. The degree of power that one individual has over another is dependent on the level of imbalance in the relationship.

Raven (1965) identified six bases of social power that people can access in order to persuade others: reward power, coercive power, informational power, expert power, legitimate power and referent power (Hogg and Vaughan, 2005):

- Reward power – a promise of reward for compliance.
- Coercive power – a threat of punishment for non-compliance.
- Informational power – a belief that the influencer has more information than oneself.

- Expert power – the certainty that the influencer has generally greater expertise and knowledge than oneself.
- Legitimate power – the belief that the influencer is recognised by a power body to make decisions and direct.
- Referent power – a respect for the source of influence, or identification with it.

THINK ABOUT THIS

How can the bases of social power be applied to nursing?

Power is implicit in all social relations including the nurse–patient relationship. Historically, nurses' approach to providing care for patients has been using the expert model of care. This approach tends to reinforce an unequal power base, allocating more power to nurses and less to patients with an expectation of patient compliance without question. Obviously this has now changed, and there is more of a partnership approach to nursing practice.

The concept of power and obedience to authority was famously demonstrated in the 1960s by an experiment undertaken by Stanley Milgram. In this study, the participants were ordinary members of the general public paid for a few days' work in the study. When they arrived at the prestigious Yale University for the study they were introduced to another 'volunteer' who was in fact a confederate of the researcher. They were told that they were taking part in a learning task and asked to draw lots to ascertain who would be the 'teacher' and who would be 'pupil'. In truth the lots were fixed: the real research participant took the role of 'teacher'. The pupil (confederate) was then taken into an adjacent room and strapped to a chair in full view of the participant (teacher). The teacher (participant) was then instructed to press a button which would give an electric shock to the pupil as punishment for every question answered incorrectly. The shocks increased in velocity from 15 volts to 450 volts, marked red for danger. The results were astounding: 26 out of 40 participants continued as instructed by the experimenter right up to the point when 450 volts were being administered and one could hear the moans and screams coming from the adjacent room.

This study demonstrates that symbols of authority can result in unquestioning obedience to authority. The fact that the study was carried out at a very prestigious university in the pursuit of scientific knowledge by lab-coated scientists demonstrates how power and status influence our decision to conform. This led to a variety of hypotheses related to the medical and nursing profession. Can the power of the nurse or medical consultant be increased by wearing a uniform – 'the white coat' – and carrying the stethoscope around the neck? Ask yourself whether this is a useful position for the practitioner or the patient/client.

THINK ABOUT THIS

As a newly qualified nurse Sara had been instilled with the ideal of client-driven practice during her training. After several weeks working on a long-term care ward for the elderly she became aware that nursing practice on this ward was not client driven. Many of the patients who asked to use the toilet were often left for long periods of time before evacuation and patients were often left in wet incontinence pads for cost-cutting reasons. What should Sara do? Should she speak to the staff nurse about her concerns?

Sara was right to show concern over the way that patients were being treated. This treatment is wholly unacceptable. Not only are nurses using excessive power to control patients wishing to use the toilet, they are also demonstrating a form of economic power over patients by leaving them in wet incontinence pads. Sara should speak to the staff-nurse over her concerns. It is important that she uses the skills that she has learnt during her training to ask questions and question the cost to patient care when asked to comply with such practice.

It is important that nurses have a proper understanding of the meaning of power and how it fits in with a client-empowering approach to nursing so that they can recognise their responsibility and regulate the exercise of power. In general practice negative power is wielded only in certain situations and when it is in a patient's best interests, for instance when there are concerns that something untoward may happen to them (Palviainen *et al.*, 2003).

THINK ABOUT THIS

How do you think these six power bases apply to the nurse–patient relationship? What about different types of patient/client - a depressed man, a psychotic woman, a middle aged man with Parkinson's disease, a child with cancer? What about other forms of relationships - the nurse–doctor relationship, for example, in a psychiatric ward, in an ENT clinic or in an operating theatre?

4.7 Conclusion

Human beings are social animals and benefit from social interaction. These social processes can influence the relationship that individual nurses have with their patients, clients and colleagues. Knowledge of this relationship can assist you with your professional practice.

4.8 Summary

- Non-verbal channels of communication are important for the good development of the patient–nurse relationship.
- Negative attitudes need to be replaced with more positive attitudes through the use of learning and direct experience.
- Cognitive dissonance is a process by which individuals are motivated to implement attitude change when they feel their cognitions are unbalanced.
- For affective persuasion Hovland *et al*. (1953) identified these steps – attention, comprehension, acceptance and retention.
- People may conform to social groups in order to validate their opinions and obtain social approval.
- Compliance to healthcare is influenced by a multitude of factors. Ley's (1981) cognitive hypothesis model of compliance identified that compliance is a mixture of patient satisfaction, understanding of the information given and ability to recall the information given during consultation.
- Obedience to authority happens in healthcare. Nurses must recognise their responsibility and regulate the exercise of power.
- Stereotyping and labelling can interfere with the delivery of personalised care.

YOUR END POINT

Answer the following questions to assess your knowledge and understanding of social processes in nursing.

1. What is cognitive dissonance?
   (a) When a person experiences inconsistencies in their cognitions
   (b) A form of non-verbal communication
   (c) An attitude towards others
   (d) A cognitive attitude towards medication
   (e) A way of understanding the person.

2. Which of the following is true?
   (a) Accurate predictions of specific behaviour can be derived from people's specific attitudes.
   (b) Attitudes formed as a result of direct experience are poor predictors of behaviour.
   (c) The more general the attitudes involved, the greater the accuracy in predicting particular behaviours.
   (d) The best conclusion is that attitudes do not predict behaviour.
   (e) None of the above.

3. Whether a teenage girl will actually undergo a vaccination is best predicted by the _____; how someone reacts to a beggar who
approaches them on the street is best predicted by the _____.

(a) theory of planned behaviour; attitude to behaviour process model
(b) attitude to behaviour process model; theory of planned behaviour
(c) theory of planned behaviour; theory of planned behaviour
(d) attitude to behaviour process model; attitude to behaviour process
model

4. A nurse who is trying to persuade someone will be better able to produce
an attitude change if he:

(a) speaks rapidly and does not deliberately set out to persuade us
(b) speaks slowly and does not deliberately set out to persuade us
(c) speaks normally and deliberately sets out to persuade us
(d) uses a lot of gestures
(e) all of the above.

5. A message that emphasises the costs of not eating breakfast is
_____; a message that emphasises the benefits of eating breakfast
is _____.

(a) generally effective; generally ineffective
(b) generally ineffective; generally effective
(c) positively framed; negatively framed
(d) negatively framed; positively framed
(e) none of the above.

Further reading

Aronson, E. (2008). *The Social Animal* (10th edn). New York: Worth/Freeman.

Eagly, A.H. and Chaiken, S. (1997). *The Psychology of Attitudes*. Fort Worth, TX:
Houghton Mifflin Harcourt.

Chesney, M. (2003). Adherence to HAART regimens. *AIDS Patient Care and STDs*, 17,
pp. 169–177.

Elwyn, G., Edwards, A., Kinnersley, P. and Grol, R. (2000). Shared decision making and
the concept of equipoise: The competences of involving patients in healthcare
choices. *British Journal of General Practice*, 50, pp. 892–899.

Rutter, D. and Quine, L. (2002). *Changing Health Behaviour*. Buckingham: Open
University Press.

Wong, N.C.H. and Cappella, J.N. (2009). Antismoking threat and efficacy appeals:
Effects on smoking cessation intentions for smokers with low and high readiness to
quit. *Journal of Applied Communication Research*, 37(1), pp. 1–20.

Weblinks

http://www.spring.org.uk/2007/11/10-piercing-insights-into-human-nature.php
PsyBlog. This blog site gives a top ten list of the major social psychology research experiments. There is also information on non-verbal communication and relationships.

http://smokefree.nhs.uk
Quit Smoking with the NHS. If reading this book has inspired you to quit smoking, or maybe you'd like to help someone else to quit, this website will help you.

http://people.umass.edu/aizen/index.html
Icek Ajzen and the Theory of Planned Behaviour. This is the website of Icek Ajzen, the developer of the Theory of Planned Behaviour. There are lots of useful diagrams and articles to help you learn more.

http://www.experiment-resources.com/stanley-milgram-experiment.html
Milgram Experiment. A video and further resources on the (in)famous Milgram experiment.

http://www.helpguide.org/mental/eq6_nonverbal_communication.htm
Non Verbal Communication Help Guide. This site provides a useful guide to interpreting others and tips on how you can use this in your relationships every day.

Chapter 5

Perception, memory and providing information

LEARNING OUTCOMES

At the end of this chapter you will be able to:

- Be aware of the impact of perception on the interpretation of situations and information

- Understand models of memory and the various memory stores

- Appreciate models of attention and their relevance to nursing practice

- Understand the impact of knowledge, satisfaction and memory on adherence

- Be aware of a number of techniques for improving your own and your patients' memory

- Be aware of some of the conditions that can result in memory loss

- Be aware of a number of factors influencing adherence to treatment; and possible interventions to improve adherence levels

- Explore various cognitive models of health behaviour and how these can be applied to nursing practice

- Be able to understand the motivational interviewing approach to changing risky behaviour.

YOUR STARTING POINT

Answer the following questions to assess your knowledge and understanding of cognition, memory and information provision.

1. The original protection motivation theory claimed that health-related behaviours are a product of, and therefore predicted by, five components. But which of the following is *not* one of these?

   (a) fear
   (b) severity
   (c) benefits
   (d) self-efficacy
   (e) none of the above.

2. Based on the theory of planned behaviour, if the important people in your life want you to cut down on the amount of alcohol that you drink, what else needs to be in place in order for actual alcohol consumption to change?

   (a) Personal belief that reducing alcohol consumption will be beneficial
   (b) Perceive self to be capable of drinking less
   (c) Subjective norms are in place
   (d) All of the above
   (e) (a) and (b).

3. Rehearsal resembles . . .

   (a) echoic memory
   (b) acoustic interference
   (c) autobiographical stories
   (d) encoding
   (e) 're-hearing' something.

4. What is a 'chunk,' in short-term memory?

   (a) a partial memory, not complete
   (b) a single organised thing or item
   (c) a 'magic number' which aids retrieval
   (d) a hierarchy
   (e) a binary 'bit' of information.

5. Cued recall involves which one of the following:

   (a) bringing information to mind in response to non-specific cues
   (b) bringing information to mind in response to specific cues
   (c) identifying information provided at test time as having been encountered previously
   (d) responding differently to previously encountered information than to new information
   (e) none of the above.

5.1 Introduction

This chapter will look at various cognitive processes – the way we perceive the world around us, the way we remember various activities and then how these processes can be combined into our professional practice. Neisser (1967) coined the phrase 'cognitive psychology' and defined it as the study of how people learn, structure, store and use knowledge. In short, this is the branch of psychology that is concerned with the study of mental states and processes such as problem solving, memory and language.

But why is this relevant to you? What use does this have in your professional practice as a nurse? Well, there are many uses and even though at first inspection hard-core cognitive psychology may not appear relevant to nursing, it probably underlies much of your professional practice. For example, patients' medication routine. How can this be enhanced? How can you as a nurse assist the patient with their medication programmes so adherence is maximised? What about dealing with the ward situation and how best to treat people? What about out in the community with people with differing needs and expectations? Cognitive psychology explores memory – what it is, what can affect it and how it can be improved. The area of perception is also important – you need to be able to take a holistic view of the patient. A community psychiatric nurse needs to be able to explore the perception of the patient, the views of the family as well as the evidence based practice you have amassed over your education. How successful the patient is in managing or recovering from an illness or state of ill-health will be determined to some degree by how much the patient retains and uses that information.

For example, look at the picture in Figure 5.1 – what do you see? You, as a student professional nurse, probably see a tool, an instrument, something that you may use frequently with your clients, or you may come across on a daily basis in your practice. But think again, what would your patient see? Would they see a tool

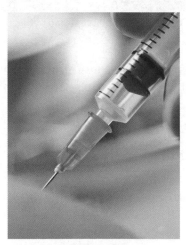

Figure 5.1 What is this?

or something useful or something common, or would they be scared? What would they expect? They may not be as used to the equipment as you are. What would their reactions be?

THINK ABOUT THIS

Consider the pictures in Figure 5.2. What do you think the psychological reactions would be to each picture from each of the following:

- a 16-year-old diabetic girl;
- a 50-year-old chronic schizophrenic;
- a six-year-old boy requiring a local anaesthetic;
- a 22-year-old woman with learning disabilities requiring a contraceptive injection?

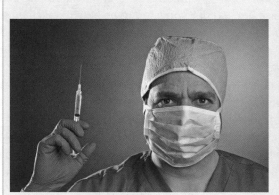
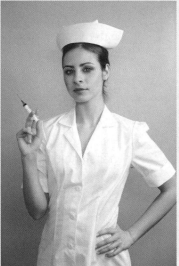

Figure 5.2 **What do you see? What does your patient see?**

This chapter will explore these mental processes and how they can influence your practice. To start with we will explore perception before moving on to memory – its definition and improvement.

5.2 Perception

Most of us will have come across the shapes outlined in Figure 5.3. But look at them again; is the one on the left a vase or two faces? Similarly the one on the right: two people may view the image as being a woman who is young, or an older woman; which do you see?

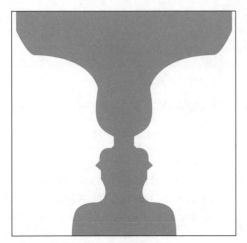
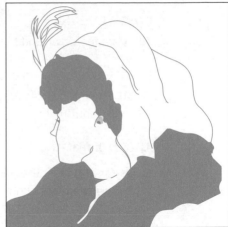

Figure 5.3 Perceptual illusions

These two illusions highlight a big issue of importance to nursing: two individuals can perceive the same stimulus in vastly different ways, and these perceptions can influence how we think and feel about that stimulus. This issue penetrates all aspects of life: for instance, to a nurse a syringe is a medical tool, an everyday object which elicits little emotional response. For a patient with a phobia of needles these same stimuli appear exaggerated and produce feelings of fear and anxiety.

The way we perceive stimuli can affect both our emotional response and our memory for that situation – 'the needle was HUGE!' Let's turn to a consideration of other factors influencing our recall of events.

KEY MESSAGE

People perceive things differently: what you see as normal and pain free may not be seen in the same way by your patients.

The visual process that has taken place when you look at those perceptual illusions in Figure 5.3 is referred to as the **top-down process**. According to Gestalt psychologists, the top-down approach is how perception works overall in that we strive to see things as a whole so that they are meaningful. In contrast to this, there is also the **bottom-up process**, which means that the shapes and colours are recognised alone and then the picture is built up. The process by which we structure the input from sensory receptors is based on the principle of perceptual organisation (Baron, 2001) which allows us to perceive shapes and forms from incomplete and fragmented stimuli. As humans we are all striving to have consistency – to fill in all the gaps.

QUICK CHECK
What are top-down and bottom-up processes?

The Gestalt principles of grouping include: figure/ground, proximity, similarity, closure and continuity.

Figure/ground

The vase shown in Figure 5.3 is an example of this tendency to pick out form. We don't simply see black and white shapes – we see two faces and a vase.

The problem here is that we see the two forms of equal importance. If the source of this message wants us to perceive a vase, then the vase is the intended *figure* and the black background is the *ground*. The problem here is a confusion of figure and ground.

Here is an example from practice:

- a nurse appears with a hypodermic needle;
- the patient will focus on the needle;
- the nurse is rather attractive (or alternatively, rather unattractive) and is carrying a needle;
- there is now confusion of figure and ground (nurse and hypodermic) and consequently less focus on the hypodermic needle.

This is not to say that in order to overcome needle phobia there should always be an attractive nurse delivering the injection! Rather it is an example where two objects (nurse/hypodermic) can swap levels of importance.

Proximity

Items or individuals which are close together in space or time tend to be perceived as grouped together. Thus, if you want your patient to associate the treatment with the nurse or practitioner, put them close together. On the other hand, if you want them to perceive two ideas as associated, present them in close proximity but not both in view. For example, you may want to hide a hypodermic needle from sight so you, the nurse, are not associated with it.

Look at Figure 5.4:

- When you look at (a) you see (a nurse + a nurse) + a bed;
- when you look at (b) you see (a nurse + a bed) + a nurse.

Similarity

Things which are similar are likely to form 'Gestalten' groups. So in Figure 5.5, on the left you probably see an X of hypodermic needles against a background of the

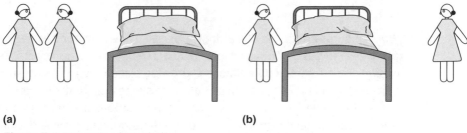

(a)   **(b)**

Figure 5.4 **Example of proximity**

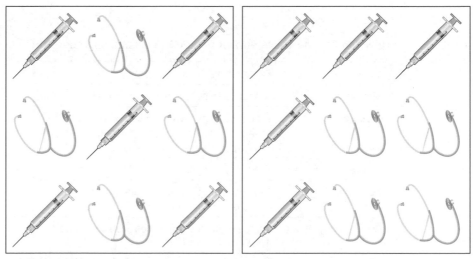

Figure 5.5 **Example of similarity**

stethoscopes; on the right you may see a square of the stethoscopes, partly surrounded by hypodermic needles. So, if we want our patients to perceive the elements of our message as belonging together we should try to give them the same shape.

Closure

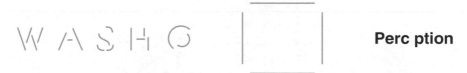

Look at this image. We can still read WASHO, see the square and read 'perception' despite the missing information. It may be that your patients often prefer to be able to complete health messages themselves and there is some evidence to suggest that, for example, health promotion messages in which the general public are required to play an active role in completion of the message is retained for longer (although there is, of course, the danger that they may complete it wrongly!).

Continuity

Where figures are defined by a single unbroken line, they tend to be seen as an entity (see Figure 5.6). This principle is of course of particular importance in graphic design. Even something as simple as drawing a squiggle to link up apparently disparate elements on a page can be helpful in suggesting to the reader that they are parts of a whole. Remember – your written messages are important and you can provide additional information to your readers by using graphic design.

Figure 5.7 shows another example of the continuity principle.

THINK ABOUT THIS

How can you use these laws of perceptual grouping in your practice?

Laws	Explanation	Your practice
Similarity	Tendency to perceive similar items as a group	
Closure	Tendency to perceive objects as whole entities despite the fact that some parts may be missing or obstructed from view	
Figure and ground	Tendency to look at the obvious figure	
Continuity	Tendency to perceive complete patterns in terms of similar shape	
Proximity	Things seen close together are seen as being associated	

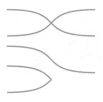

1 When you see figure 1, you are much more likely to see it as consisting of two lines like 1a, rather than of the two shapes like 1b.

1a This is the Gestalt principle of continuity.
1b A single unbroken line is likely to be seen as an entity.

Figure 5.6 **The Gestalt principle of continuity**

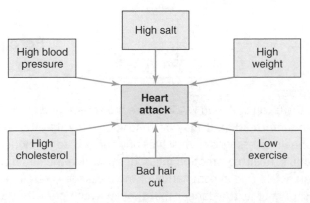

Figure 5.7 **Continuity principles – items can be suggested to be linked even if bizarre!**

KEY MESSAGE

There are several perceptual laws that can be incorporated into your practice.

QUICK CHECK

Name the Gestalt principles of grouping.

5.3 Memory

A cognitive process that plays a significant role in the day-to-day practice of nurses and patients is our memory. The importance of memory permeates all aspects of our lives – we would be little without a functioning memory. If we explore our professional activities then we can see we need to have good memory. We need to recall the names of our colleagues and patients, we need to remember what we have learned at university. We need to remember our patient's diagnosis, how to treat them, our daily routines, what has been discussed with a patient and how they are going to progress. It also has an important role for patients – understanding, decision making and their ability to follow the treatment regime.

In this section the nature and processes of memory, as we currently understand it, will be outlined, and the implications of this knowledge on nursing practice will be discussed. Common problems in encoding and retrieving knowledge will be explored and the causes and impact of common patterns of memory loss will be outlined.

KEY MESSAGE

Memory is what makes us human and is involved in all our daily activities.

What is memory?

Memory is commonly accepted to be made up of three central processes: encoding, storing and retrieving information. **Encoding** refers to the process whereby sensory information is transformed into a representation (e.g. some kind of chemical memory trace) suitable for storage. **Storage** refers to the process by which sensory information is retained within the memory system. **Retrieval** refers to the process whereby stored information is recovered. This is also known as 'recall' or 'remembering'.

KEY MESSAGE

Memory is made up of encoding, storing and retrieving information.

What has this got to do with nursing?

As mentioned earlier, an important part of a nurse's role is to communicate with the patient, to help them understand their diagnosis, its implications on their daily lives, and the treatment options available to them. The way in which this is communicated to the patient will affect the way in which this information is coded, stored and subsequently recalled. It also has an impact on the patient's ability to cope with the behavioural and emotional consequences of their condition and on treatment decision making. Similarly, there is an abundance of research to suggest that forgetting is of central importance in non-adherence to treatment plans and, in turn, this may affect patients' overall recovery and quality of life.

How is memory structured?

Most psychologists agree that there are at least two distinct memory stores – short-term memory (STM) and long-term memory (LTM). Trying to remember a telephone number for a few seconds is a popular example of short-term memory as it illustrates two central features: STM doesn't hold very much information (it has a limited capacity); and it doesn't last for very long (it has a limited duration). LTM on the other hand can (in theory) last for a lifetime. For example, you might recall your childhood memories or a gift you received on your birthday five years ago.

> **KEY MESSAGE**
>
> Memory has both a short-term and a long-term component.

Memory stores

Atkinson and Shiffrin (1968) developed one of the first systematic accounts of the structures and processes involved in human memory. The 'multi-store model' or 'dual process theory' proposes that memory consists of three distinct stores: a sensory store, STM store and LTM store – see Figure 5.8. According to the model, information from the environment is received by the sensory store. A small fraction of this information is attended to where it is processed further by STM. In turn, and only after sufficient rehearsal, information processed in the STM store is

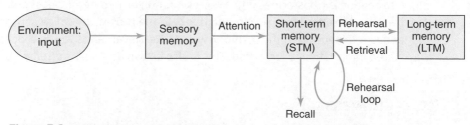

Figure 5.8 **Multi-store model of memory**

transferred to LTM. If rehearsal does not occur, then information is forgotten. Thus the more the information is rehearsed, the stronger the memory trace.

Evidence supporting the distinction between short-term and long-term memory comes from Glanzer and Cunitz (1966). They carried out an experiment in which they presented participants with a list of words and asked for free recall (a memory test in which the words can be recalled in any order). When free recall occurred immediately after the list was presented there was evidence for a **recency effect**, meaning that participants typically recalled those items from the end of the list first and got more of these correct. There was also evidence of a **primacy effect**, meaning that the first few words in the list were also well remembered. Poorest recall was for those items in the middle portion of the list.

THINK ABOUT THIS

Think about providing information on medical treatment to an individual with the following: anxiety disorder, moderate learning disabilities, angina, Parkinson's disease. What sort of aspects of memory should you take into account?

It was argued that the recency effect reflected retrieval from STM, whereas the primacy effect reflected retrieval from LTM. Glanzer and Cunitz tested this hypothesis by employing an interference task (counting backwards) between learning and recall. The idea was that if the recency effect does demonstrate STM, by preventing rehearsal the effect should disappear. Indeed, Glanzer and Cunitz found that counting backwards for only 10 seconds virtually eliminated the recency effect, but otherwise had no effect on recall. Further evidence for separate stores comes from studies investigating capacity, duration and encoding.

KEY MESSAGE

You can use primacy and recency effects in your practice: important information should be presented either at the start or end of a consultation.

QUICK CHECK

Draw the multi-store model of memory.

Sensory memory

Sensory memory is a basic form of storage, which retains very brief, literal copies of sensory information needed for STM. It is modality specific (i.e. information is held in the form in which it was received), has a large capacity for information (although only a fraction of this information is actually processed) and functions outside of awareness. According to the multi-store model there is a separate store for each sensory register, i.e. vision, hearing, smell, taste, etc. However, most research has concentrated on the **iconic store** (visual store) and the **echoic stores** (auditory store).

THINK ABOUT THIS

How can your knowledge of sensory memory assist with your practice?

5.4 Attention

There is a considerable overlap between the areas of memory and attention. For example, Broadbent's (1958) filter theory of selective attention was in many ways the main precursor of the multi-store model. Broadbent argued that sensory stimuli from the environment gain access in parallel to a sensory buffer. One of the inputs is then selected (filtered) on the basis of its physical characteristics (e.g. familiarity, comprehensibility), while the other stimuli remain in the sensory buffer store for later processing. If the stimuli are not processed they are filtered out. This filter is needed to prevent the limited capacity of STM from becoming overloaded. Once past the filter the information is processed thoroughly.

QUICK CHECK

What inputs into the sensory buffer?

Information received within sensory memory can decay rapidly so it is important for the nurse to ensure that the patient is attending to the health information being provided. It is also important that the information is familiar and intelligible to prevent it being filtered out. Understanding health information can be problematic when the information is complex or new; thus information should be conveyed to the patient using everyday examples and avoiding medical jargon.

The number of distractions a patient encounters can also explain how much information is attended to. Within the hospital setting there are many distractions such as busy wards and high levels of background noise; not to mention internal distractions such as pain, fear or anxiety. Using a slightly higher tone of voice and expressing interest while talking (Cherry, 1966), referring to the patient by name and acknowledging internal distractions are simple yet effective techniques which will focus the patient's attention.

Information that is delivered in a variety of different formats is more likely to be attended to. A simple way of delivering information in different formats is to use written material to complement verbal information. Indeed research suggests that complementing verbal information with written material can increase patients' attention, enhance comprehension and improve recall. Researchers have also highlighted the importance of using other aids to complement verbal information. For example, Scott *et al.* (2006) recommended aids such as consultation tapes and summary letters. The use of pictures in addition to verbal information has also proved helpful when recalling information, particularly for those who have low literacy skills (Houts *et al.*, 2006).

> **THINK ABOUT THIS**
>
> What distractions were there in the environment when you were talking to your last patient? What influence did these distractions have on them and their recall of information? What could you do about it?

Short-term memory

The capacity of STM has been investigated using span measures. This is an assessment of how much information can be stored in memory at any one time. In a review of studies Miller (1956) found that the capacity of STM was seven plus or minus two items and that this was irrespective of whether the items were numbers, letters or words. As seven words will always contain more than seven letters, one might think that a person should remember fewer words than letters. However, in his article Miller illustrated how **chunking** (i.e. integrating units of information) can be used to extend the capacity of STM and explain this phenomenon.

> **THINK ABOUT THIS**
>
> When revising information for a recent examination, how could you use chunking to aid your revision?

For example, seven letters or seven numbers each constitute seven chunks. Likewise, seven words would also represent seven chunks, despite containing considerably more letters. Whenever we reduce a large amount of information into a smaller amount we are chunking: this not only increases the capacity of STM but also increases the likelihood that the information will be stored for longer. It also denotes a form of encoding, by imposing a meaning on otherwise meaningless letters or numbers. Obviously what constitutes a 'chunk' will depend on your personal experience. For example, 'NHS' is one chunk as long as you are familiar with the National Health Service. If you are not familiar with this then the abbreviation 'N H S' would constitute three chunks.

> **KEY MESSAGE**
> **The shorter the chunks, the easier is it to remember the information. Chunking can help!**

TIME TO TRY

Quickly read through the list of letters below, then cover the list and try to write the letters down in the correct order.

S	A	V	A	O
R	E	E	E	G
U	R	S	Y	A
O	O	D	N	S
F	C	N	E	R

How many did you remember in the correct order? The likelihood is that you remembered about seven letters (plus or minus two). Now look at the letters again starting with F (bottom left-hand corner) and read upwards until you get to S and then drop down to C until you get to A and so on. Did you recognise the chunks? If you did you should have remembered all of the letters.

F O U R S C O R E A N D S E V E N Y E A R S A G O

This should give you 'four score and seven years ago'.

Making use of chunking techniques during a consultation can significantly improve patients' recall of health information. A nurse can 'chunk' a verbal consultation by breaking up information with open questions. This will not only ensure that the patient understands the previous chunk of information, but will also highlight aspects of the consultation that the patient may not have understood. When chunking information it is important to consider that patients are more likely to remember the first thing and the last thing that has been stated (this is the primacy/recency effect discussed earlier in this chapter); thus nurses should endeavour to provide the most important 'chunk' of information at the beginning and/or end of the consultation.

Rote rehearsal (also known as maintenance rehearsal) is a technique which involves repeating information over and over again out loud. This technique is useful when communicating information that is complex or new. One way of applying this technique would be to ask the patient to repeat what has been said as well as referring back to important information throughout the consultation.

> **KEY MESSAGE**
> Get your patient to repeat the information – this can aid memory for the information.

Audio or video recording the consultation can also act as a method of rehearsal and in turn facilitates patient recall. For example, Thomas *et al.* (2000) found that approximately 80 per cent of patients who listened to an audio recording of their consultation rated it as useful or very useful. Likewise, Liddell *et al.* (2004) found that providing patients with an audiotape reduced misunderstandings and improved comprehension. What's more, 24 per cent of patients reported hearing information not attended to during the consultation.

As we have just noted, rehearsing information can improve memory recall. Rehearsal or repetition seems to require some kind of inner speech, whereby we 'say' the information either overtly or mentally again and again to keep it circulating within STM. This suggests that STM may encode information acoustically.

According to Gibson *et al.* (2002), patient confusion often arises because health information is too complex or lacks clear relevance to the patients' situation. Thus, In order to prevent patient confusion the nurse should ensure that health information is brief, simple and linked to patient goals (British Thoracic Society and Scottish Intercollegiate Guidelines Network, 2003). Attributing meaning to health information can lead to greater recall.

> **THINK ABOUT THIS**
> What memory techniques can you use to improve memory for information in your patients?

> **KEY MESSAGE**
> Brief, simple and categorised information aids memory.

Long-term memory

LTM is often categorised into episodic and semantic memory (Tulving, 1972), explicit and implicit memory (Graf and Schacter, 1985), and declarative and procedural knowledge systems (Cohn and Squire, 1980). Episodic memory contains memories about specific experiences or events occurring in a particular place at a particular time. Semantic memory on the other hand contains memory for factual information about the world. Typical examples of semantic memory include knowledge about language, how to calculate percentages and the dates of the Second

World War. 'Explicit memory is revealed when performance on a task requires conscious recollection of previous experiences' (Graf and Schacter, 1985: 501). The memory tests discussed earlier in this chapter (e.g. free recall) all involve the use of explicit memory. In contrast, 'Implicit memory is revealed when performance on a task is facilitated in the absence of conscious recollection' (Graf and Schacter, 1985: 501). A typical example of implicit memory would be being asked to write a list of the countries you have visited – you know the names of the countries not because you were instructed to learn them, but because you have learned them in the natural course of events. Finally, explicit memory depends largely on the declarative knowledge system, whereas implicit memory depends largely on the procedural knowledge system. Declarative and procedural knowledge systems are related to Ryle's (1949) distinction between 'knowing that' and 'knowing how'. An example of declarative knowledge is *knowing that* Paris is the capital of France, whereas an example of procedural knowledge is *knowing how* to ride a bicycle.

QUICK CHECK

What are the main categories of LTM?

The capacity of LTM is very large and generally considered to be unlimited; yet the truth is that no one really knows how much information LTM can store. It is likely, however, that there must be a physical limit in terms of the actual brain cells available, but it seems unlikely that we will ever reach this upper limit. Table 5.1 outlines the features of different forms of memory.

How long does LTM last? Because of the difficulties in measuring LTM, a precise estimate cannot be given; however, we do know that the elderly never lose their childhood memories and that many skills such as such as riding a bicycle are never forgotten. Therefore, in theory, information can be held in LTM for several years, which may in fact span the individual's entire lifetime. Bahrick *et al.* (1975) produced a simple but clever demonstration of LTM using photographs from high-school year books. They asked 392 ex high-school students of various ages to recall the names of people in their class. Researchers also showed them a set of photographs and asked them to identify individuals. Even after 34 years participants were able to name 90 per cent of photographs of their classmates, supporting the idea that LTM does indeed store information for a very long time.

Table 5.1 Comparing short- and long-term memory

	Sensory memory	*Short-term memory*	*Long-term memory*
Duration	¼ to 2 seconds	Up to 30 seconds	Unlimited
Capacity	Large	7 +/– 2 items	Unlimited

5.5 Information presentation

Two theories which are particularly applicable when looking at how information is presented are the levels of processing theory and schema theory. These will be briefly outlined and recommendations for practice will be discussed in relation to their suggestions.

Schema theory

A theory that can explain a number of errors in the memory process, both at the encoding and retrieval stages, is schema theory. A schema is a mental script, which guides individuals and influences how they perceive and interpret events around them based on previous experiences. When we receive information, we locate it within a schema. Schema theory discusses the way in which information or memories are organised. The theory suggests that our knowledge of people or events is stored in an elaborate network based on our pre-existing knowledge of that event or person. Basically, individuals have slots in which to store information about different things, for example you may have a professional experience slot, a hospital slot and a treatment slot holding all the information you have about that person, situation or object. When no direct knowledge about that subject is available it is filled with anecdotal evidence from friends or the media, and this then provides a base from which to predict or interpret events involving that subject.

These structures aid us to carry on our everyday lives by providing a structure from which to understand and deal with the complex world around us; they also save a lot of cognitive effort. There are several types of schema, each of which assists us in different activities;

- person schemas (e.g. patient)
- self-schemas (e.g. about you)
- role schemas (e.g. nurse)
- event schemas (e.g. hospital).

This information is important since these structures may impact negatively on memory for medical information. The pre-existing information you or your patient holds can impact on how information is interpreted and consequently on behaviour. For example, stereotypes (see Chapter 4) are a simple cognitive framework for dealing with whole groups of people, which can be perpetuated by inferences made from nursing uniforms (Alford *et al.*, 1995).

QUICK CHECK

List the different forms of schema.

THINK ABOUT THIS

What is the general stereotype of nurses? How can this influence how you behave or are treated?

Launder *et al.* (2005) also suggest that this can cause problems when patients have pre-existing ideas about their medication, illness or their treatment and are given more (accurate) information. Moreover, information can be distorted to fit the current schema. The nurse should ensure that preconceived ideas and beliefs are explored fully with the patient before new information is provided, which also enhances patient-centred care (Price, 2006).

KEY MESSAGE

Information you give to your patient may be distorted based on what the patient thinks you are trying to tell them and their existing information.

Levels of processing model

Another theory that can add to our understanding of patients' memories for health information is the levels of processing model (Craik and Lockhart, 1972). According to this model, it is the depth at which information is processed that is important in terms of how it is stored and subsequently recalled. Processing information according to its meaning produces stronger, longer-lasting and more elaborate memory traces than processing information according to its sound (phonemic processing) or physical appearance (shallow processing). Referring back to the initial models presented, short-term memory is that which is processed at a shallower level (e.g. acoustically), whereas long-term memory lasts longer as it is remembered in terms of its meaning. This therefore removes the need for separate storages, with information existing on a continuum in terms of its depth of processing.

This theory tells us of two methods when rehearsing information; rehearsing material by simple rote repetition, or maintenance rehearsal, is classified as shallow. Rehearsing material by exploring its meaning and linking it to semantically associated words is called elaborative rehearsal and is classified as deep.

So, how can we use this information? How can this improve our own memory, and how can we use it with our patients? Providing health information within the context of the patient's everyday life is one way of enhancing meaning; this can be done, for instance, by linking prescribed medication to the patient's everyday routine. This theory also explains the success of mnemonic techniques for enhancing recall, a method discussed later in the chapter. Furthermore, we also need to explore (at each level) the understanding of the information to ensure that deep processing has occurred. There are a number of other methods for improving memory and we will explore these in more detail later in this chapter.

5.6 The role of cues

We have all had the experience of going somewhere, be it upstairs, to the kitchen, to a particular patient and then when getting there, forgetting why we had come, so we backtrack either physically, returning to where we were, or mentally, what was I thinking about that reminded me to do this? These are great examples of the role of cues in memory recall. It may be that you have experienced situations in which a patient was doing well with their treatment plan but upon returning home failed to adhere to the plan and returned to hospital.

THINK ABOUT THIS

How can you use cues in your practice to get the following individuals to take their medication:

- a 45-year-old with chronic schizophrenia;
- a 24-year-old with epilepsy;
- a person with pre-senile dementia;
- a 16-year-old with diabetes?

It is important to provide patients with cues to act that not only occur within the hospital setting but can be transferred to the home setting. So what is it that cues do that works so well? Levels of processing theory would suggest that cues are the meaning to which meaningless activities such as doing an exercise or taking a pill are attached. By putting this information within a meaningful situation such as a daily routine, it is recalled better. If we look back at schema theory, cues can be explained as the activation of a network of information for which the action is a part. Hence, Park *et al.* (1992) report on how external cues can be used with older adults to improve their memory for treatment and hence medication adherence.

> **KEY MESSAGE**
>
> Cues can aid recall and improve adherence to treatment.

5.7 The role of perceived importance

It sounds obvious, but information is less likely to be remembered if the patient considers it to be unimportant: for example, if a patient does not understand the implications of not taking their medication at particular intervals then they are less likely to remember and subsequently do not adhere to this routine. The role of importance in memory encoding and recall has been displayed in a number of research studies. Kessels (2003), based on the work of Ley (1979), highlights the importance of information in memory. If the importance of the information is stressed then there is an improvement in adherence.

> **KEY MESSAGE**
>
> Stressing the importance of a message can improve adherence to treatment.

5.8 Mnemonic aids

'I' before 'e' except after 'c'. Mnemonics are a well-known way of aiding memory and work by pairing a meaningless stimulus, such as the type of drug used to treat a particular condition, with a meaningful stimulus, something already in the long-term memory, such as a daily routine or journey. If we return to the levels of processing theory, you can see that this technique works by attaching meaning to new information providing a deeper memory trace and as such results in a more memorable piece of information. There is a lot of support for the success of these techniques, particularly in teaching children with learning disabilities (Goll, 2004) or those with emotional or behavioural disturbance (King-Sears et al. 1992). Some further examples of mnemonic aids are presented in Table 5.2.

> **THINK ABOUT THIS**
>
> Consider the various topics you need to revise for your study. Think of some mnemonics to help you do this.

Table 5.2 Mnemonic use in nursing practice

Mnemonic principle	Definition	Example in practice
Elaboration and the keyword mnemonic	Converting names into meaningful words or even making words active.	The 12 cranial nerves: 'Oh Oh Oh, To Touch And Feel A Girl, Very Sexy & Hot.'* Olfactory nerve (I) Optic nerve (II) Oculomotor nerve (III) Trochlear nerve (IV) Trigeminal nerve (V), subdivided into Abducens nerve (VI) Facial nerve (VII) Vestibulocochlear nerve (VIII) Glossopharyngeal nerve (IX) Vagus nerve (X) Accessory nerve (XI), Hypoglossal nerve (XII)
Association	Giving meaning to a word or name which then must be attached to something.	Take for instance the need to take certain medication on specific days. You could use the name of the drug as a clue, say amoxicillin, a must until the weekend. If the name of the pill is too long or complex then using the colour or shape of the medication is another memory trick. Yellow pills could be bananas, blue could be blueberries, etc.
Story system	Advantage over the link system is that the flow of the story will allow the remainder of the list to be retrieved whereas the link system will lose all the information if one link has been lost.	I walked into the house and saw my bowl of fruit – my yellow bananas – and then I went into the kitchen and got my blueberries . . .
Loci system	Based on the principle of mentally positioning things to remember in a well-known room.	Visualise your tablets in your bathroom so you remember them always.
Rhyming word peg	Rhyming meaningful words or numbers with established words.	To the tune of 'Row, row, row your boat' to assist in remembering the characteristics of DNA: **We love DNA,** Made of nucleotides, A phosphate, sugar and a base, Bonded down one side. Adenine and Thymine, Make a lovely pair, Guanine without Cytosine, Would be very bare.

*There is a ruder version of this one!

5.9 Compliance, adherence and concordance to treatment

To date in this chapter we have considered various cognitive processes – perception, attention and memory – from a very technical perspective. However, these come together when the patient is attempting to follow information from the nurse or other healthcare practitioner. This used to be termed 'compliance', but was retermed 'adherence' during the 1980s. However, both terms suffer from the implication that it is an authoritarian relationship – the nurse or healthcare professional telling the patient what to do. Consequently, the term 'concordance' is now used within the literature to indicate more of a partnership approach: 'The patient being an equal partner, supporting the ethos of shared decision-making between patient and health professional rather than more traditional paternalism' (Weiss and Britten, 2003).

KEY MESSAGE

Compliance, adherence and concordance refer to the same thing, but concordance is the most appropriate term: it emphasises the partnership between the patient and the nurse.

Therefore, compliance and adherence refer to the cooperation of a patient in following medical advice about treatment, whereas concordance takes into consideration the needs and desires of the patient (Snowden, 2008). Another distinction that has to be emphasised is intentional versus unintentional non-adherence. For example, on some occasions the patient will not follow the advice given since it was not explained properly, or it has been forgotten. In this case, it can be classified as unintentional non-adherence. In contrast, there are occasions when the patient makes an active choice not to take the medication as instructed.

THINK ABOUT THIS

Why would a patient choose not to take their medication as indicated?

There are low levels of adherence to many forms of medication and this has a significant impact on the expenditure of the health service. Snowden suggests that non-adherence costs the NHS some £6.8 billion in the UK alone. However, more important on an individual basis is the potential significant impact on the patient. For example, estimates of non-adherence to medication for unipolar and bipolar disorders range from 10–60 per cent with a median rate of 40 per cent (Lingam and Scott, 2003). Similarly, some 20–70 per cent of headache sufferers are not using medication optimally and 40 per cent non-adhere to appointment keeping (Rains *et al.* 2006). In cross-sectional studies published from 1980 to 2001, around 18–22 per cent of renal graft recipients were found to be non-adherent to immunosuppressants (Gremigni *et al.* 2007).

It is not just in physical health that there are issues, but also in mental health. Cramer and Rosenheck (1998) report that in people with schizophrenia the average rate of non-adherence is 42 per cent and McAllister-Williams *et al.* (2006) suggest that low adherence is becoming a major concern for individuals with bipolar disorders.

Thus, non-adherence results in a number of negative consequences: reduced positive recovery on the part of the patient, high frustration levels and wasted time on the part of the healthcare professional, and significant costs to the health service. In the next section of this chapter we will look at the possible causes of non-adherence and will then turn to possible psychosocial interventions for improving adherence levels.

KEY MESSAGE

Non-adherence can be costly both to the taxpayer and the individual patient.

5.10 Causes of non-adherence

A useful model for exploring non-adherence is based on the work of Phillip Ley who presented a cognitive model of compliance (1981, 1989). According to this cognitive hypothesis, patient adherence can be predicted by patient satisfaction, understanding, and memory (recall) (see Figure 5.9).

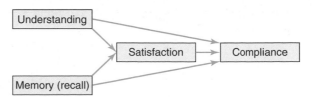

Figure 5.9 The cognitive hypothesis model of compliance

THINK ABOUT THIS

How do you think you can influence (either positively or negatively) patient satisfaction?

In terms of patient satisfaction there are three elements: (i) the cognitive aspect - satisfaction with the amount and quality of the information provided by the healthcare professional; (ii) the affective aspect - the extent to which the patient feels that that the healthcare professional listens, understands and is interested; (iii) the behavioural aspect - the patient's evaluation of a healthcare professional's competence in the consultation (Wolf *et al.*, 1978).

QUICK CHECK

What are the components of non-adherence according to the cognitive hypothesis model?

However, the major focus of this chapter is on the other two factors: understanding and memory. Any setting where treatment is being offered can be a highly anxious and distressing environment (remember the perceptual point we highlighted at the outset of this chapter). Consequently you will want to reduce anxiety and concern. Hence, if treatment is completed in a more relaxed setting (e.g. at home) then there is a better chance of any recall.

There are different ways in which the nurse can provide instructions for treatment and the method will influence how likely a patient is to remember them. For example, the more oral and written information you can provide a patient, the more likely you are to enhance their adherence (McDonald *et al.*, 2002). This is because information that is received by more than one sense is more likely to be registered within memory and retained for a longer period of time (see above). However, there are also many other methods that can help improve recall of information and some of these are presented in Table 5.3 and the impact of these improvements in Table 5.4.

KEY MESSAGE

Written information can improve understanding and adherence.

Table 5.3 Guidelines for improving information recall

Guideline	Example
Keep information simple	Do not over-complicate with medical jargon – use everyday language.
Important information at the start (primacy) or at the end (recency)	Provide the most important information at either the start or the end of the conversation.
Divide the information into chunks	'I am now going to talk about your diagnosis, and now your prognosis, and now your treatment . . .'
Explain and ensure information is meaningful	Relate to the individual patient – make it meaningful for them and ensure that it will fit in with their particular situation.
Ensure understanding	Ask questions to test understanding.
Stress the important message	'This is of central importance . . .'
Repeat information	And repeat, and repeat . . .
Be specific rather than general	'Lose 2lbs in weight' rather than 'Lose some weight'.
Follow up	Phone the patient or discuss at the next consultation to ensure understanding.

Table 5.4 Effectiveness of these techniques for increasing recall

Technique	Control (i.e. without the technique)	With the technique
Primacy	50	86
Stressed importance	50	65
Simplification	27	40
Explicit categorisation	50	64
Repetition: by practitioner	76	90
Repetition: by patient	76	91
Use of specific statements	16	51
Mixture	55	75

THINK ABOUT THIS

How could you improve adherence to treatment in the following:

- overweight male on a weight reducing regime;
- person with asthma on an exercise regime;
- male with heart failure requiring considerable medication;
- person with kidney failure?

5.11 Cognitive models of health behaviour

The cognitive hypothesis model has been useful and indicates some key factors involved in adherence to treatment. However, it does not really address some fundamental concerns about the individual patient – their feelings, concerns and cognitions concerning their health and illness. In order to address this, further models – the social cognition models – have been developed. These models are 'concerned with how individuals make sense of social situations' (Conner and Norman, 1996:5). These models are the subject of this section. They have been used to explain why people adhere (or don't) to treatment, but also to whether they will engage in health protective behaviour (e.g. going for screening tests or stopping drinking).

> **KEY MESSAGE**
>
> Cognitive models of health behaviour have been a major focus of attention in psychology. They have been used to explain why people engage in health promoting, health protecting or health damaging behaviours.

The earliest models were based on the belief that behaviours were a result of a rational weighting of the potential costs and benefits of that behaviour and that the behaviour is a result of rational information processing of these costs and benefits (spot the potential problem already?). Several models have been proposed as explanations for health behaviour and behaviour change.

The health belief model

The **health belief model (HBM)** was one of the first and best-known models (Rosenstock, 1974; Becker, 1974) developed in order to predict preventative heath behaviours – see Figure 5.10. It has also been used to describe the behavioural response to treatment in patients with both acute and chronic illnesses.

The HBM makes a series of predictions about behaviour and suggests that they are a result of a set of core beliefs. The original core beliefs are the individual's perception of:

- susceptibility to illness (e.g. 'My chances of getting cancer are high');
- severity of the illness (e.g. 'Cancer is a serious illness');
- the costs involved in carrying out the behaviour (e.g. 'Quitting smoking will be stressful');

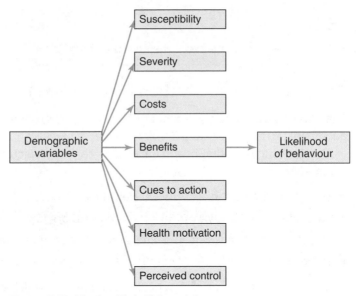

Figure 5.10 **The health belief model**

- the benefits involved in carrying out the behaviour (e.g. 'I will be able to run up the stairs');
- cues to action, which may be internal (e.g. some non-specific symptoms) or external (e.g. health education information/leaflets).

The model suggests that the likelihood of a behaviour occurring is related to these core beliefs. Consequently, the HBM can be used to predict whether a behaviour will occur or not. The original HBM has been updated and improved with 'health motivation' added to reflect an individual's readiness to be concerned about health matters (e.g. 'I am concerned that not stopping smoking will seriously damage my health').

THINK ABOUT THIS

How can the HBM be used to deal with various health promoting behaviours?

Recognising that the HBM had several components that needed to be further developed, and some factors that needed to be included, prompted researchers to refine this model and in light of these studies the protection motivation theory (PMT) was developed.

QUICK CHECK

What are the components of the health belief model?

The protection motivation theory (PMT)

The PMT was developed by Rogers (1975, 1983) who expanded the HBM to include additional factors (see Figure 5.11).

The PMT suggests that health behaviours can be predicted on the basis of four components:

- severity (e.g. 'Heart disease is a serious illness');
- susceptibility (e.g. 'My chances of getting CHD are high');
- response effectiveness (e.g. 'Doing some exercise would improve my health');
- self-efficacy (e.g. 'I am confident that I can engage in physical exercise').

These components predict behavioural intentions which are related (although somewhat tenuously) to behaviour. The PMT considers that severity, susceptibility and fear are part of the threat appraisal (external factors) and response effectiveness and self-efficacy are related to coping (internal factors).

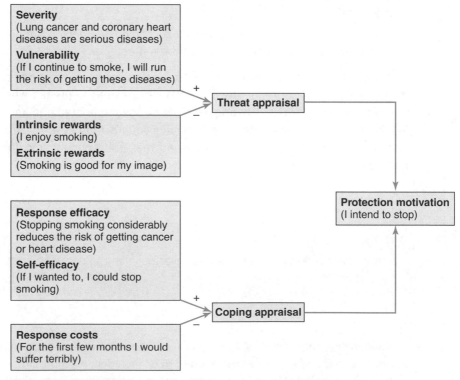

Figure 5.11 Protection motivation theory

Source: Based on Stroebe, 2000.

THINK ABOUT THIS

How would you use the PMT to increase the chances of a patient attending a breast screening clinic?

QUICK CHECK

What are the components of the PMT?

5.12 Social cognition models

The two models thus far described have been further developed and revised in order to overcome some of the criticisms levelled against them. In particular, the models have been refined to include a role for the social context of the behaviour and not simply rely on the individual's cognitions or attitudes. Not surprisingly these models have been called 'social cognition models' (as opposed to 'cognition models').

Theory of reasoned action

The theory of reasoned action (TRA) was developed by social psychologists in the 1970s and has been used extensively to examine predictors of behaviours (Fishbein, 1967; Ajzen and Fishbein, 1970; Fishbein and Ajzen, 1975). The TRA was an important model as it was one of the first to place the individual within the social context.

KEY MESSAGE

The theory of reasoned action places the individual within a social context.

The TRA suggests that behavioural intention is a product of an individual's attitude towards performing the behaviour and of subjective norms. Each of these factors has further elements – see Figure 5.12.

So, for example, a person's attitudes towards the behaviour will be a consequence of the likelihood of that behaviour being associated with a positive outcome. Hence, an individual's attitudes towards starting exercise is a function of the perceived likelihood with which physical exercise is associated with certain consequences, such as being healthier and fitter, and the evaluation of these perceived consequences (i.e. Are they positive? Are they worth the effort?).

The other element to the model is subjective norms and this includes two components: normative beliefs and motivation to comply. Normative beliefs are the beliefs

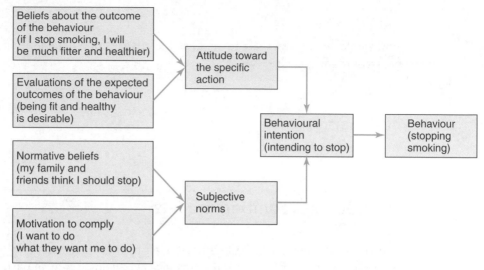

Figure 5.12 **Theory of reasoned action**

Source: Wolfgang Stroebe, *Social Psychology and Health*, 2nd edn, 2000. Reproduced with the kind permission of Open University Press. All rights reserved.

held by us about how people who are important to us expect us to behave. Hence, subjective norms are a product of both normative beliefs and motivation to comply.

QUICK CHECK

What are the key components of the TRA?

Theory of planned behaviour (TPB)

The TRA was developed by Ajzen and colleagues into the theory of planned behaviour (Ajzen, 1985, 1988) – see Figure 5.13.

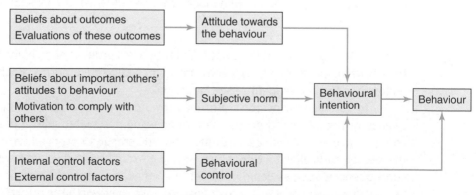

Figure 5.13 **Theory of planned behaviour**

Source: Jane Ogden, *Health Psychology*, 3rd edn, 2004. Reproduced with the kind permission of Open University Press. All rights reserved.

The TPB suggests that behavioural intentions (i.e. to engage in a particular practice – to behave in a certain manner) are a consequence of a combination of several beliefs:

- **Attitudes towards a behaviour**: this comprises a positive or negative evaluation of a particular behaviour and beliefs about the outcome of the behaviour (e.g. 'Exercising is fun and will improve my health').

- **Subjective norms**: these are composed of the perception of social norms and pressures to perform a behaviour and an evaluation of whether the individual is motivated to comply with this pressure (e.g. 'My husband is important to me and he will approve if I lose weight and I want his approval').

- **Perceived behavioural control**: this is an important component and suggests that the individual can carry out the particular behaviour considering both internal (e.g. skills, abilities and information, 'I can play five-a-side football and I know where to join a club') and external (e.g. 'I can make the Friday night when the football sessions are on'). Obviously both of these relate to previous experiences and behaviour.

THINK ABOUT THIS

How would you use the TRA and TRB to increase the chances of an individual using a condom when she has sex with her partner? In particular, how would you increase perceived behavioural control?

5.13 Strategies for changing risk behaviour

So far in this chapter the various models that have been devised to predict people's behaviour have been outlined and explored and the value of these to nursing demonstrated. However, of course, one of the important areas for any heathcare professional is in altering an individual's maladaptive behaviour to positive health-promoting behaviour. This will be the focus of the final section of this chapter. In particular, the concept of motivational interviewing will be developed and discussed (Miller and Rollnick, 2002) which was based on the stages of change model (Prochaska and DiClemente, 1982).

One of the most influential psychological models that has been used in behaviour change has been the 'transtheoretical model of change' or 'stages of change' (Prochaska and DiClemente, 1982). The model suggests that change proceeds through six stages summarised in Figure 5.14 and Table 5.5 on page 171. Importantly, relapse can occur at any stage, and can mean that the individual goes back to the very first stage. It is not a linear model of simple progression from one stage to another and then relapse means that you simply revert to the previous stage: you can revert to *any* previous stage.

Pre-contemplation	Contemplation	Determination/preparation	Action	Maintenance	Relapse/recycle
	Fence	0–3 Months	3–6 Months	Over 6 months	
No: denial	Maybe: ambivalence	Yes, let's go: motivated	Doing it: go	Living it:	Start over: ugh!!

Figure 5.14 Stages of change model

KEY MESSAGE

Always find out where your individual patient is on the stages of change model as this will determine your intervention.

QUICK CHECK

What are the stages in the stages of change model?

THINK ABOUT THIS

What intervention strategies would you recommend to a smoker in each of the following stages:

pre-contemplation; contemplation; preparation; action; maintenance?

The stages of change model has been used extensively to promote health and assist individuals in quitting smoking. This model is important because it allows professionals to identify where individuals are in their behaviour and then develop appropriate interventions (whether these be computer or media based, community or individual based, pharmacologically or psychologically based).

If, for example, an individual smokes and has no intention of giving up (i.e. is in the pre-contemplation stage), the intervention to be developed will be different to that of the individual that is preparing to give up (i.e. is in the contemplation stage) or has started the process (i.e. is in the action stage). In the first case our obligation should be to try to get quitting into the person's thought processes. We want to try to get the individual to consider giving up smoking – we want to shift them from the pre-contemplation stage to the contemplation stage. The most common method in this approach is a simple consciousness-raising exercise: increasing information about the problem and how it can affect the individual concerned. So at this stage

Table 5.5 Stages of change – definitions and description

Stage	Definition	Description
Pre-contemplation	No intention of change	The person changing the behaviour has not been considered: the person may not realise that change is possible or that it might be of interest to them.
Contemplation	Intention to change	Something happens to prompt the person to start thinking about change – perhaps hearing that someone has made changes or something else has changed resulting in the need for further change.
Preparation	Intention to change soon and plans of action have been made	Person prepares to undertake the desired change – requires gathering information, finding out how to achieve the change, ascertaining skills necessary, deciding when change should take place. May include talking with others to see how they feel about the likely change, considering the impact change will have and who will be affected.
Action	Making changes	People make changes, acting on previous decisions, experience, information, new skills and motivations for making the change.
Maintenance	Working to maintain behaviour and prevent relapse	Practice required for the new behaviour to be consistently maintained, incorporated into the repertoire of behaviours available to a person at any one time.

it would simply be a case of getting them to realise that smoking is health damaging and that it can affect them individually and then spelling out the individual health problems. This example demonstrates that interventions have to be tailored to the individual's position in the cycle.

On a scale of 1 to 10 how certain are you that you want to change your smoking behaviour?

1	2	3	4	5	6	7	8	9	10
Not certain at all									Very certain
Pre-contemplation			Contemplation			Action			

Figure 5.15 Readiness ruler for assessing stage of change of a smoker

On a scale of 1 to 10 how confident are you that you *want* to change your smoking behaviour?

1	2	3	4	5	6	7	8	9	10
Not confident at all									Very confident

Figure 5.16 Confidence ruler for assessing an individual smoker

> ### KEY MESSAGE
> **Interventions have to be specific to the individual's stage of change.**

Interventions to help people quit smoking, based on the stages of changes model, usually incorporate two key elements. Firstly, it is necessary to identify accurately an individual's stage of change (or readiness to change), so that an appropriate intervention can be designed and applied. Secondly, the stage of change needs to be reassessed frequently, and the intervention modified in light of this assessment. In this way, stage based interventions evolve and adapt in response to the individual's movement through the stages.

The first task that we have to do is identify what stage the individual smoker is at. This is not as difficult as it sounds and can be completed using a simple 'readiness ruler' as indicated in Figure 5.15 along with a confidence ruler (see Figure 5.16) which can assist the practitioner in planning the intervention and the support that will be required. (Note that these rulers can be adapted for any behaviour.)

Motivational interviewing

On the basis of the stages of change model a whole series of interventions can be devised, described and implemented. Motivational interviewing has as its goal the simple (some would say!) expectation that increasing an individual's motivation to consider change rather than showing them how to change should be the important step. If a person is not motivated to change then it is irrelevant if they know how to do it or not. However, if a person is motivated to change then the interventions aimed at changing behaviour can begin.

Motivational interviewing (MI) is a technique based on cognitive-behavioural therapy which aims to enhance an individual's motivation to change health behaviour. The whole process aims to help the patient understand their thought processes and to identify how these help produce the inappropriate behaviour, and how they can be changed to develop alternative, health-promoting behaviours.

KEY MESSAGE

A person must be motivated to change in order to start their change process.

Motivational strategies include components that are designed to increase the level of motivation the person has towards changing a specific behaviour. It is important to note that the motivation is specific to one behaviour – so being motivated to quit smoking does not simply transfer to being motivated to reduce alcohol consumption. Some of the essential skills for motivational interviewing are presented in Table 5.6.

Table 5.6 **Key skills for motivational interviewing**

Skill	*Comment*
Use open-ended question	Encourage the client to do most of the talking: 'What are your concerns about smoking?'
Use reflective listening	Reflect back change talk in a statement: 'I have the shakes in the morning' to 'You are a little concerned about the shakes in the morning . . .'
Use affirmation	Use to build rapport: 'You are right to be concerned about having unprotected sex.'
Summarise	Link together and reinforce what has been discussed: 'You are concerned that your smoking may cause lung cancer.'
Reframe or agree with a twist	Address resistance by reinterpreting: 'My wife nags me to change my diet' to 'It sounds like she really cares about your health.'
Emphasise personal choice	Reinforce that it is the client's choice to change their behaviour.
Evocative questions	
Increasing confidence	Use open questions to evoke confidence: 'How might you go about making this change?'
Confidence ruler	Use the ruler to ask: 'What would it take to score higher?'
Strengths and successes	Review obstacles and how the client has overcome them.
Reframing	'I've tried three times to quit and failed' to 'You have had three good attempts already and are learning new skills'.
Prompt coping strategies	Ask for potential obstacles and putative coping strategies.

However, before we get to the questions we need to assess readiness to change and this is usually completed using a 'readiness to change' ruler. This is exactly what is says! Hence, the nurse would ask the patient, 'On a scale of 1 to 10 how ready are you to make the change?' (whether this be change to diet for somebody with diabetes, quitting smoking or reducing alcohol intake and so on). On this basis you could decide whether the patient was in the pre-contemplation stage (probably scoring 3 or below), the contemplation stage (scoring 4–6) or the action stage (7 or above). On this basis you would then tailor your intervention (see Figure 5.17).

THINK ABOUT THIS

How would you use motivational interviewing to increase an individual's likelihood of quitting smoking?

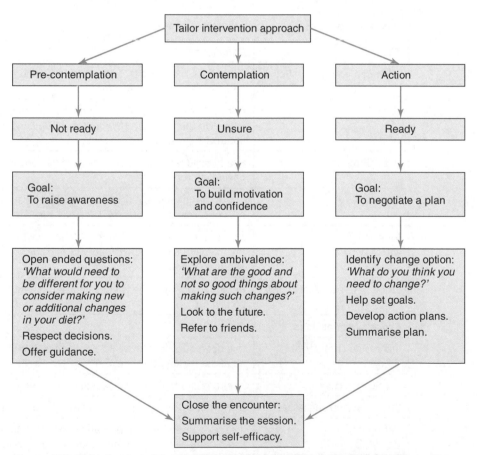

Figure 5.17 Tailoring your intervention strategy according to an individual's readiness to change

5.14 Conclusion

Perception, attention and memory are all elements in healthcare practice and can impact on your patients' and clients' behaviour. This may help explain adherence to treatment and possible ways of improving this.

5.15 Summary

- People perceive items and individuals differently.
- Gestalt principles of grouping including similarity, proximity, continuity, closure and figure/ground and can be used in nursing care practice.
- Memory is made up of three components: encoding, storing and retrieving information.
- STM and LTM are different memory stores.
- Recency and primacy effects are important in conveying and remembering information.
- Too much information in the environment can lead to distraction and an inability to recall.
- Chunking and mnemonics can improve recall.
- The cognitive hypothesis suggests that understanding, memory and satisfaction influence levels of adherence/compliance.
- The HBM is based on susceptibility to illness, severity of illness, costs and benefits of carrying out the behaviour along with cues to action.
- The protection motivation theory (PMT) suggests that health behaviours can be predicted on the basis of severity, susceptibility, response effectiveness, self-efficacy and fear.
- The theories of reasoned action/planned behaviour are social cognition models which are based on attitudes towards a behaviour, subjective norms and perceived behavioural control.
- A particular method for developing behaviour is motivational interviewing which aims to increase an individual's motivation to alter their own behaviour.

YOUR END POINT

Answer the following questions to assess your knowledge and understanding of cognition and information provision.

1. Information about how to approach familiar situations such as a day on the ward, organising your studies or ordering in a restaurant is organised into knowledge structures referred to as _____

   (a) sketches
   (b) schemes
   (c) episodes
   (d) schemas
   (e) loops.

2. When some participants read an ambiguous passage about a woman, Sarah, in a nurse's office, which psychological factor reduced the accuracy of their recall of the information from the passage?

   (a) imagined memories of the event
   (b) expectations about recalling the passage at a later time
   (c) expectations about Sarah's condition
   (d) pre-existing knowledge about people named Sarah
   (e) the number of times they read the passage.

3. The improved recall of items presented at the end of a consultation compared to the middle of a consultation is referred to as the _____

   (a) last rehearsed effect
   (b) recency effect
   (c) delayed effect
   (d) limited capacity effect
   (e) none of the above.

4. Based on the stages of change model developed by Prochaska and DiClemente (1982), if a person notices that she has been coughing a lot recently and begins to think about stopping smoking over the next six months, she would be at which stage of making behavioural changes?

   (a) pre-contemplation
   (b) contemplation
   (c) preparation
   (d) action
   (e) maintenance.

5. According to Ajzen's (1985) theory of planned behaviour, behavioural intentions are influenced by:

   1. The objective norms regarding the behaviour.
   2. The attitude towards the behaviour.

3. Perceived control over performance of the behaviour.
4. All of the above.
   (a) 1 and 2
   (b) 2 and 3
   (c) 1 and 3
   (d) 4
   (e) none of them

Further reading

Atkinson, R.C. and Shiffrin, R.M. (1968). The control of short-term memory. *Scientific American*, 225, pp. 82–90.

Bohner, G., Moskowitz, G.B. and Chaiken, S. (1995). The interplay of heuristic and systematic processing of social information. *European Review of Social Psychology*, 6, pp. 33–68.

Floyd, D.L., Prentice-Dunn, S. and Rogers, R.W. (2006). A meta-analysis of research on protection motivation theory. *Journal of Applied Social Psychology*, 30(2) pp. 407–429.

Gillibrand, R. and Stevenson, J. (2006). The extended health belief model applied to the experience of diabetes in young people. *British Journal of Health Psychology*, 11, pp. 155–169.

Levine, J.M., Resnick, L.B. and Higgins, E.T. (1993). Social foundations of cognition. *Annual Review of Psychology*, 44, pp. 585–612.

Navon, D. (1977). Forest before trees: The precedence of global features in visual perception. *Cognitive Psychology*, 9, pp. 353–383.

Zimmerman, G.L., Olsen, C.G. and Bosworth, M.F. (2000). A 'stages of change' approach to helping patients change behaviour. *American Family Physician*, 61, pp. 1409–1416.

Weblinks

http://www.memoryarena.com/resources
Memory Resources. This site contains links to the latest memory journal articles.

http://www.umbc.edu/psyc/habits/content/the_model/index.html
Transtheoretical Model of Behaviour Change. This site provides details of how health promotion techniques can be designed using the transtheoretical model.

http://www.mindtools.com/memory.html
Mind Tools. This site contains hints and tips for improving your own memory.
Why not have a go!

http://www.patientadherenceroi.com
Patient Adherence. This site contains lots of useful articles on patient adherence
to treatment.

Chapter 6

Stress and stress management

LEARNING OUTCOMES

At the end of this chapter you will be able to:

- Define stress

- Evaluate the various models of stress

- Describe the link between stress and ill-health

- Review how people cope with stress

- Explore how you can employ stress management techniques for your patient.

YOUR STARTING POINT

Answer the following questions to assess your knowledge and understanding of stress and stress management.

1. Being impatient, irritable, always in a hurry, and fixated on deadlines are traits associated with:
   (a) latency stage fixation
   (b) type A Personality
   (c) type C personality
   (d) type B Personality
   (e) oral stage fixation.

2. As you peek through the door of the ward where you are just about to start, you notice that one of your colleagues is being berated by a drunken youth. Your first stress response is:
   (a) alarm and mobilisation
   (b) plateau
   (c) resistance
   (d) exhaustion
   (e) fixation.

3. On your way to work one morning, you get stuck in traffic and you are 45 minutes late for your shift. This is an example of:
   (a) a background stressor
   (b) a personal stressor
   (c) an uplift
   (d) learned helplessness
   (e) a depressive episode.

4. You tell a patient that he must take a prescribed medicine twice daily to cure his infection. The patient eventually discards the medicine for a 'home remedy' suggested by his grandmother. This demonstrates:
   (a) subjective well-being
   (b) objective well-being
   (c) civil disobedience
   (d) rational non-adherence
   (e) none of the above.

5. Selye describes the general adaptation syndrome as proceeding in the following order:
   (a) alarm reaction, resistance, exhaustion
   (b) alarm reaction, exhaustion, resistance
   (c) exhaustion, resistance, alarm reaction
   (d) resistance, alarm reaction, exhaustion
   (e) none of the above.

6.1 Introduction

It is important to recognise that all of us suffer from stress at some point in our lives. We can all probably recognise the symptoms of it – the thoughts that flash through our minds, the physiological reactions (e.g. increased heart rate or sweating palms), or the emotional consequences (the fear and the anxiety). We all know what it is and how it affects us. But can we define it? What is stress all about? This is important since whilst everyone experiences stress there are some people that probably face greater stressors than others. This may be you, as a nurse, or it may be your patient, or it may be one of your health professional colleagues. You need to be able to recognise stress and be able to cope with it successfully.

Furthermore, we all can probably list the health consequences of stress – considerable stress results in heart attacks, doesn't it? We are all aware of the reports of top bankers or high-flying business people that suggest they are just heart attacks waiting to happen. But we also know that stress can result in milder forms of illness – both physical and psychological. When we are under constant stress the likelihood of us developing a cough or a cold is higher. When some are under considerable stress then there is the threat of a 'nervous breakdown'. So, stress obviously exists and it affects our lives at all levels, resulting in both mild and severe illnesses. But what exactly is it, and what can be done about it?

As a nurse you will need to understand stress and stress management strategies to benefit both you and your patients. In this chapter we will explore how stress can lead to both physical and mental health problems and why this is of direct relevance to you and your patients.

KEY MESSAGE

Stress is an everyday phenomenon that affects us all.

THINK ABOUT THIS

List all the potential stressors of:

- working in an acute mental health ward;
- working on an A&E ward during a multiple road traffic accident (RTA);
- working in a hospice for terminally ill children;
- being a student nurse and coping with university studies and practice;
- working with a difficult line manager.

6.2 What is stress?

The first thing that we have to do, of course, is try to define what stress is. This shouldn't be a difficult thing to do, surely? Probably all of us use the term in our daily lives and we all know what the consequences of it are. However, when you stop and consider this question you begin to appreciate that it may not be as easy as you first thought.

THINK ABOUT THIS

Write down all the terms that you associate with stress. Discuss these with your colleagues – have they come up with any different terms?

On completing this exercise you may end up with a number of different terms or phrases. Masse (2000) posed this same question to members of the general public and he came up with more than 2000 terms associated with the concept of stress. This may, of course, lead to some confusion – for example, when you talk to your patient about 'stress' and they talk about 'strain' or being 'worried' or 'all tensed up' – but you are both talking about the same concept. However, this difficulty is relatively easily overcome – we can usually appreciate when somebody is under stress and we know what they are really talking about.

The next question can really highlight some individual differences – what exactly causes stress? If you ask a couple of colleagues what causes stress for them, you will probably come up with a range of different factors.

WHAT CAUSES STRESS?

Ask a couple of friends to list all of the things that they find stressful on a table similar to the one below.

You	Friend 1	Friend 2

Have you found a couple of things that you share and have in common or are they all completely different? On the one hand, you might have all listed similar activities such as exams, going to the dentist or giving a verbal presentation in front of a large audience. However, there might also be some activities that you cannot agree on. For example, although some of you may consider giving a presentation to an audience stressful, some of you may consider it a 'thrill' or exciting rather than being a negative experience. Similarly, some might consider exams to be useful because they allow us to demonstrate our knowledge and expertise in a subject.

> **KEY MESSAGE**
>
> **Stress means different things to different people.**

6.3 Models of stress

Stress has been explained in many different ways, although these can essentially be reduced to three different categories:

- stress on the outside;
- stress on the inside;
- the interaction between the inside and the outside, i.e. between the person and the environment.

Stress on the outside

Stress is there on the 'outside' – it is something that happens to us whether this is a big event (e.g. a death in the family) or a minor daily irritant (e.g. not being able to find a parking space at the local supermarket). These 'stressors' can be chronic (e.g. caring for somebody with an illness), acute (e.g. taking an exam or going for a screening test), a daily hassle (e.g. traffic jams) or life events (e.g. getting married or divorced).

> **KEY MESSAGE**
>
> **There are certain life events that are more stressful than others.**

Most people can identify with these forms of stressors. Holmes and Rahe (1967) tried to make this approach more systematic and devised a life event scale or the social readjustment rating scale (SRRS). This scale weighted each of a series of events according to how stressful each one was. The most stressful, as rated by the respondents, was the death of a spouse which scored 100, whilst marriage was rated 50, and Christmas 12 (see Table 6.1).

Table 6.1 **The SRRS**

Event	Weighting	Event	Weighting
Death of a spouse	100	Change in number of arguments with spouse	35
Divorce	73	Mortgage/major loan	31
Marital separation	65	Foreclosure of loan	30
Jail term	63	Change in work	29
Death of family member	63	Child leaving home	29
Personal injury/illness	53	Trouble with in-laws	29
Marriage	50	Outstanding personal achievement	28
Being fired	47	Wife starts/stops work	26
Marital reconciliation	45	School starts/ends	26
Retirement	45	Change in living conditions	25
Change in health of family member	44	Trouble with boss	23
Pregnancy	40	School/house move	20
Sex difficulties	39	Minor loan	17
Gain of new family member	39	Change in sleeping habits	16
Business readjustment	39	Vacation	13
Change in financial state	38	Christmas	12
Death of a close friend	37	Minor violations of the law	11
Job change	36		

Source: Based on Holmes and Rahe (1967)

THINK ABOUT THIS

What sort of stresses and strains do you have combining your university work with working in practice? Can you and your friends come up with some items that you think are particularly stressful for you and your colleagues? Rank them in order of stress for each of your friends.

What about patients? What sort of stressors can you imagine them facing when they come into contact with the healthcare system?

Many studies have found an association between these stresses, their severity and the onset of illness. But of course, there are problems with the assessment of 'life events': what you find stressful may not be as stressful to your friends or colleagues (e.g. some people enjoy exams and others don't). Some people will experience a great deal of life events at certain times of their lives but although these may be troublesome most people do not collapse. So this cannot be the complete picture and there must be other elements to stress.

THINK ABOUT THIS

Close your eyes and try to imagine this scene. You are walking into an Accident and Emergency unit after being told on the phone that your partner is critically ill following a road traffic accident. How do you feel? Describe your feelings.

QUICK CHECK

What is the most stressful form of life event? What is the relationship between life events and stress?

Stress on the inside

This is one of the earliest models of stress: it focuses on the body's reaction (Kemeny, 2003) and is known as the physiological **general adaptation syndrome (GAS)** identified by Selye (1956). The type of bodily responses we experience when under stress (e.g. increased heart rate, increased blood pressure, increased respiration and so on) are part of the 'flight or fight' syndrome and are part of preparing the body for action as mediated through the nervous and endocrine system (see Figure 6.1).

Despite criticisms of the GAS model it still remains influential and most up-to-date models of stress have attempted to integrate some of the ideas from the GAS.

KEY MESSAGE

Stress can have an adverse affect on the body's physiology.

QUICK CHECK

Name the three stages of the general adaptation syndrome (GAS) model.

The interaction between the inside and the outside

Lazarus and Folkman (1984, 1987) proposed an alternative model of stress that took into account psychological variables. Lazarus argued that stress involved a

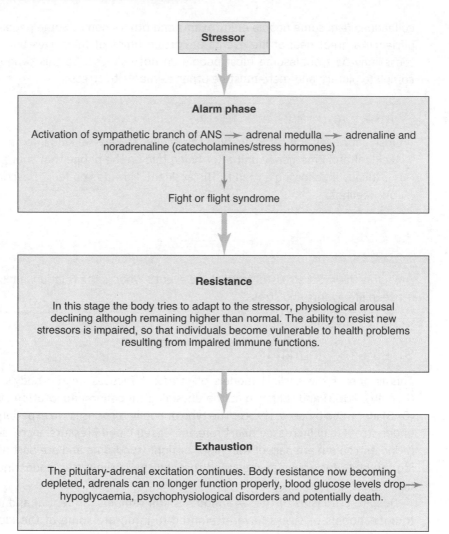

Figure 6.1 Model of the GAS

transaction between individuals and their external world, and that a stress response was elicited if an individual *perceives* a potentially stressful event as being stressful. Hence, in this model it is only if the event is perceived as stressful that it is stressful. Consequently, this model deals with those people that find exams stressful (i.e. they perceive them as stressful) and those that do not (i.e. they perceive them as fun!).

Appraisal of the event happens twice (see Figure 6.2). During *primary appraisal* the event is appraised as to whether it poses a threat, is positive or is neutral. For example, waking up to a snow storm may be seen as positive (because you will not have to go to work or to university), neutral (because you will be able to carry on with whatever you intended to do whether it was snowing or not) or it might be negative (i.e. stressful because you have an important meeting that you have to get to).

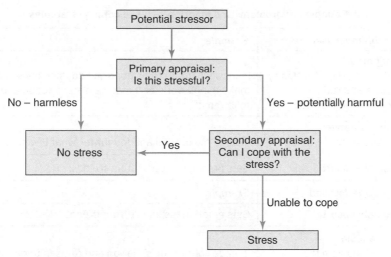

Figure 6.2 **Interactional model of stress**

If the situation is perceived to be threatening then *secondary appraisal* occurs – can we cope with the threat? Hence, secondary appraisal involves an individual evaluating their coping strategies. Can I cope with this stress, and if so how? If on the basis of these forms of appraisal the individual considers the situation to be threatening and lacks the resources to cope effectively with it then they will experience some form of stress.

KEY MESSAGE

Stress is an interaction between the person and the environment.

6.4 Coping with stress – how to do it

So how do people cope with stress? According to Lazarus and Folkman (1984), coping has two main functions: it can alter the problem causing the stress (i.e. problem-focused coping) or it can regulate the emotional response to the problem (i.e. emotion-focused coping). A number of different coping mechanisms have been described to lie within these broad categories (Folkman and Lazarus, 1988) and some of these are presented in Table 6.2.

QUICK CHECK

What are primary and secondary appraisal?

Table 6.2 **Examples of problem- and emotion-focused coping strategies**

Problem-focused	Example
Planning: analysing the situation to arrive at solutions to correct the problem	'I knew what had to be done so I doubled my efforts to make things work' or 'I made a plan of action and followed it'.
Confrontative: assertive action taken	'I stood my ground and fought for what I wanted'.
Social support	Gets practical support from friends.
Emotion-focused	Example
Social support	Gets emotional support from friends.
Distancing: detaching from the situation	'I made light of the situation and refused to get too serious about it' or 'I went on as if nothing had happened'.
Escape-avoidance: thinking wishfully about the situation	'I wished that the situation would go away or somehow be over with' or 'I hoped a miracle would happen'.
Self-control: moderating own feelings	'I tried to keep my feelings to myself' or 'I kept others from knowing how bad things were'.
Accepting responsibility: acknowledging own role in the problem while trying to put it right	'I criticised myself' or 'I made a promise to myself that things would be different next time'.
Positive reappraisal: creating a positive meaning from the situation	'I changed or grew as a person in a good way' or 'I came out of the experience better than I went in'.

THINK ABOUT THIS

Using the table of coping strategies, how would you advise a person to cope with:

- an injection;
- their relative being sectioned under the Mental Health Act;
- their child being diagnosed with a life limiting condition;
- their father dying;
- their colleague failing an exam?

It should also be pointed out that coping differs in its success ratings for different people – what one person uses may not be suitable for another. It also has to be highlighted that some coping methods (e.g. drinking large amounts of alcohol) may be useful for reducing stress, but increases other problems (see later).

QUICK CHECK

List some problem-focused and emotion-focused coping strategies.

What does this mean to me?

The model has three important implications. Firstly, no event can be characterised as stressful (or unstressful) *per se*. Any situation can be appraised by one individual as stressful but not by another. It is important to recognise that something that we may take as an everyday occurrence may be stressful for others. We therefore have to consider this when dealing with patients, clients and members of the general public on a daily basis. Something we view as mundane and routine may be considered stressful and worrying.

Secondly, since the model is based on an individual's thought processes (i.e. cognitive appraisal) then it is susceptible to changes in mood, health and other mental states. An individual may interpret the same event in different ways depending on the way they are feeling. Thirdly, a stressful response may be experienced irrespective of whether the situation is recalled, experienced or simply imagined. Hence, imagining going to the dentist can be considered by some to be just as stressful as actually going.

THINK ABOUT THIS

What daily activities are you involved in that you consider routine and (almost) boring that you think others would consider stressful? How do you think you could best reduce the stress on others?

6.5 The link between stress and health

There are a number of potential indicators of stress and these may be broadly categorised as psychological and physiological (see Table 6.3). Obviously the psychological factors can lead to poor mental health and in chronic cases poor physical health (Yehuda and McEwen, 2004).

A number of illnesses have been linked to stress and continue to be so by both the general public and healthcare professionals (Lundberg, 2006). Surveys have

Table 6.3 Psychological and physiological consequences of stress

Psychological	Physiological
Unease	Persistently elevated BP (leading to clinical hypertension)
Apprehension	
Sadness	Indigestion
Depression	Constipation or diarrhoea
Pessimism	Weight gain or loss
Listlessness	CHD
Lack of self-esteem	Gastric problems
Negative attitudes	Menstrual problems
Short temper	
Fatigue	
Poor sleep	
Increased smoking	
Increased alcohol	

indicated that stress and related conditions form a massive group of work-related ill-health conditions (Jones *et al.*, 2006). It is estimated that work-related stress, depression or anxiety affects over half a million people in the UK with an estimated 12.8 million lost working days due to these work-related conditions in 2003/04. This means that, on average, almost a month per year is lost per affected case and makes stress the largest contributor to the overall estimated annual days lost from work-related ill-health (HSE, 2005).

Evidence also suggests that most of those reporting work-related heart disease (some 66,000 people) ascribed its cause to work stress. These reports have mainly concerned the mental health effects of stress. However, there are also suggestions, and in some cases evidence, of a link between stress and physical illness (e.g. Cohen, 2005; Lundberg, 2006). This has come from a number of sources and stress has been implicated in a number of different conditions including heart disease (Clark, 2003), cancer, HIV/AIDs and other infectious disorders (Langley *et al.*, 2006).

KEY MESSAGE

Stress leads to physical and mental ill-health.

Coronary heart disease (CHD)

Overall, the evidence does suggest that there is a link between stress and coronary heart disease – the greater the stress, the greater the chance of experiencing a heart attack. Coronary heart disease is the physical condition for which there is the most comprehensive evidence of a link with stress (Bunker *et al.*, 2003; SIGN, 2007) and one which most members of the general public, including those that have had a heart attack, believe to be linked (Clark, 2003). Research suggests that **psychosocial** variables may increase the risk of CHD by three or four times, a similar increase to that as a result of biological variables (e.g. hypertension and dyslipaemia).

Breast cancer

Many studies have reported that there is a relationship between life events and the onset of breast cancer, although others suggest that the studies are flawed. Lillberg *et al.* (2003) prospectively investigated the relationship between stressful life events and risk of breast cancer. The results indicated that life events, particularly divorce/separation and death of a close relative, were linked to the onset of the cancer. So again, although there is some academic debate about the quality of the studies conducted, there does appear to be a link between the onset of breast cancer and stressful events (Garsson, 2004).

HIV/AIDS

There is some evidence that stress can lead to a progression of HIV/AIDS (Leserman, 2003). Evans (1997) suggested that the more severe the life stress experienced, the greater the risk of early HIV disease progression. For example, they reported that the risk of disease progression was doubled for every incident of severe stress in the preceding six-month period.

Infectious diseases

Obviously stress does not cause infectious diseases. However, it can reduce the body's defences against viruses by impairing the immune response. Cohen *et al.* (1998) reported that those who had experienced stress of a long duration, primarily as a function of unemployment or family conflict, exhibited a substantially greater risk of developing a cold. They also reported that participants with low numbers of social ties were four times more likely to develop a cold than those with a higher number of ties (Cohen, 2005).

Other physical conditions

A number of other conditions, for example MS, rheumatoid arthritis, type I (insulin dependent) diabetes, systemic lupus erythemastosus, bronchial asthma and irritable bowel syndrome, have been reported as being adversely affected by stress. However, for most of these conditions the evidence is equivocal. Although the role of stress in the primary aetiological process is limited, the stronger evidence suggests that the stress process can aggravate the severity of these disorders and are involved in their exacerbation (Schneiderman *et al.*, 2005; Yehuda and McEwen, 2004).

KEY MESSAGE

Stress has been linked to the development and progression of a number of physical disorders.

THINK ABOUT THIS

How does this information help you as the nurse? What does it mean for you as a professional?

Stress and mental health

Stress can adversely affect mental health in a number of different ways. It is reported by many as a precursor to many mental health problems, but it can also exacerbate any current conditions. The most common mental illnesses associated with stress are anxiety and depression. The most common symptoms of anxiety include: palpitations, headache, backache, breathing difficulties, feeling tense, keyed up, on edge, worrying about things and panic attacks. The common symptoms of depression include lack of concentration at home and work, impaired sleep, feeling depressed, bouts of crying, poor appetite, sexual difficulties, decreased energy and fatigue.

THINK ABOUT THIS

Next time you talk to someone who has suffered a recent illness – whether it be major (e.g. a heart attack) or minor (e.g. an infection), or a physical health (e.g. heart attack) or mental health problem (e.g. a 'breakdown') – discuss with them whether they can link this to any major life events. Use the Holmes and Rahe scale (see page 184).

They probably can - but what does this mean? Does it mean that the stressful event caused the physical illness, or that people just try to attribute blame? This is one of the problems with retrospective recording of the stressful events – memories differ and there is a tendency to attribute the onset of an illness to a memorable event – even if the two were not related. Consequently, the best type of studies are prospective, where recording of life events are taken before any ill-health onset.

6.6 How does stress affect health?

The research evidence indicates that there does appear to be a relationship between stress and health status. Explaining how these difficulties come about has led to a number of explanations. Physiological reactions to stress play a part but other routes worthy of further investigation are through the immune system (psychoneuroimmunology) and through changes in behaviour.

The three routes from stress to illness are therefore:

- direct physiological reactions;
- psychoneuroimmunology;
- behavioural change;

Route 1: Physiology

The way stress affects health has been related to three different physiological pathways: the neural pathways, the hormonal pathway and the immune systems.

Route 1a: The nervous system

The **nervous system**, which includes the **central nervous system** (CNS) - the brain and spinal cord - as well as the peripheral nervous system (all other neurons), controls the body's reaction to stress. The peripheral nervous system is divided into both the somatic nervous system (responsible for movement and senses) and the autonomic nervous system (ANS) which serves the involuntary muscles and internal organs. There are two branches to the ANS - the sympathetic division which deals with bodily excitation and the expenditure of energy, and the parasympathetic division concerned with reducing bodily activity and restoring energy.

From this brief description it should be possible to see how the concept of Cannon's fight or flight can be interpreted in light of this physiological reaction, especially the sympathetic division of the ANS. Hence, when an individual is under stress the sympathetic division of the ANS innervates the adrenal medulla (part of the adrenal gland) and this results in the release of two chemicals, known as catecholamines: adrenaline (sometimes called epinephrine) and noradrenaline (or norepinephrine). These two neurotransmitters mobilise the body's resources, preparing it for fight or flight. For example, increasing the cardiovascular activity (heart rate, stroke volume and force of contraction), shifting the flow of blood to the muscles rather than digestion or the skin, widening the airways, speeding the rate of breathing and increasing the volume of air intake into the lungs are some of the many reactions. These bodily reactions can be mapped onto the reactions of stress, which are highlighted in Table 6.4.

The repeated occurrence of these responses is one way in which stress can impact on health. For example, the repeated cardiovascular activation could lead to permanent damage to the arteries and veins and thereby cause elevated blood pressure.

QUICK CHECK

List the physiological consequences of stress and how these manifest themselves as symptoms.

Table 6.4 **Physiological reactions to stress and potential symptoms**

Physiological reaction	Potential symptoms
Increase in heart rate	Rapid or irregular heartbeats
Increase in respiration rate	Hyperventilation or some form of asthma
Adrenaline released	Increase in heart rate
Noradrenaline released	Raised blood pressure
Muscle tightening	Tension headache, tense muscles, insomnia, fatigue, loss of concentration
Change in blood flow/circulation	High blood pressure, cold hands, upset stomachs, migraine, pre-ulcerous/ulcerous conditions, increased colitis, constipation and sexual dysfunction
Senses heightened	Emotional irritability, poor impulse control, reduced communication abilities
Increased perspiration	Dehydration
Imbalance in hormone	Frequent infections, auto-immune disease
Saliva consistency change	Dry mouth

Route 1b: The hormonal system

The hormonal (or endocrine) system consists of a number of glands throughout the body which secrete hormones in times of stress, although at a much slower rate than the neurotransmitters described above. For this reason they are mainly associated with chronic stressors (rather than the acute stressors that influence the nervous system). The hormones are carried in the bloodstream to various parts of the body where they act on the target organ (either directly or indirectly). These hormonal reactions are much slower to act than the neurotransmitters but also have a longer lasting effect.

One major hormonal pathway through which stress exerts its effects is the adrenocorticotrophic hormone (ACTH). The anterior pituitary produces ACTH when it is stimulated by the hypothalamus. ACTH is released into the bloodstream and acts upon the outer area of the adrenal gland causing it to produce a group of hormones – the corticosteroids. These regulate the blood pressure and hence this demonstrates one mechanism whereby hormonal transmitted stress can exert a negative effect.

Route 1c: The immune system

The immune system protects us from infection and illness and consists of a series of coordinated responses to protect the body by defending it against invasion by antigens. Immune reactions involve two main types of response. In the first the immunity involves the action of a special white blood cell called the T-cell, which kills invading micro-organisms. In the second, special chemicals known as antibodies or immunoglobulins are released into the bloodstream which attach themselves to the antigen and destroy it. A third type of cell involved in the immune response is known as a phagocyte which envelops and devours foreign substances.

Route 2: Psychoneuroimmunology (PNI)

The term psychoneuroimmunology was first coined by Adler (Adler, 1981; Adler *et al.*, 2001) and involves the study of the interactions between behaviour, neural and endocrine functions and the immune process. Early research indicated that there was a link between stress and the immune system and this was first observed in bereaved spouses. The reports suggested that bereaved spouses have a weaker immune system than those in continuing relationships.

Later Kiecolt-Glaser *et al.* (1987) reported that a sample of women who had recently divorced or separated had a poorer immune system than a control group (Kiecolt-Glaser *et al.*, 2005) and those that had a positive marital environment had a better immune response (Heffer *et al.*, 2004). This means that those who got divorced had a weaker immune system than those who had not. Women who were more attached to the marriage showed a greater response than those who showed less positive memories of the marriage. Similar findings were reported for men who had been separated or divorced. Similarly, Kiecolt-Glaser and Glaser (1992) found immune suppression in carers of Alzheimer's patients. Those caring for people with a dementing illness had a poorer immune system and hence were more prone to disease.

Workman and Lan Via (1987) explored the immune system in students undertaking an exam (an acute stressor) and noted a weakening in the immune system from a baseline prior to the exam, to during the exam and then after the exam. The studies have also found that the whole immune system appears to be affected, and this appeared to be the case even when behavioural factors such as lack of sleep, diet and drug use were controlled for. Hence, this study, amongst others, suggests that those students undertaking exams had a poor immune response – hence they were at a greater risk of developing infectious disorders.

Route 3: Changing behaviour

THINK ABOUT THIS

Think about the last time you were under exam stress. Did you change your behaviour? Did it become healthier or unhealthier? Did you, for example, smoke more, drink more or eat the wrong things?

It is often the case that when a person is under stress they change their behaviour and try to cope with this stress in a number of different ways. That is, coping strategies are used in order to reduce the stress (as we have seen before with the transactional model of stress). However, some of these coping strategies may be successful in reducing an individual's stress but may, ironically, actually result in an increased health risk (see Table 6.5).

Table 6.5 How do people cope (badly) with stress?

	What the research suggests	Problems, problems . . .
Smoking	People smoke more when they are stressed, and are more likely to start and restart under episodes of stress. Studies have reported that higher levels of smoking more cigarettes are linked with higher levels of stress (Heslop *et al.*, 2001).	Smoking kills you! It leads to a host of health problems including cancer, heart disease and breathing problems.
Alcohol	The tension reduction theory suggests that people drink alcohol because of its tension reducing properties (Cappell and Greeley, 1987). This theory is supported by evidence of a relationship between negative mood and drinking behaviour which suggests that people are more likely to drink when they are depressed or anxious.	Too much alcohol can lead to liver and cardiac problems along with a whole host of other physiological and social consequences.
Eating	Cartwright *et al.* (2003) found that there was some evidence to support the myth of comfort eating. The report found that those under stress were more likely to eat fatty foods than fruit and vegetables and more likely to snack unhealthily. Furthermore the authors report: '. . . a dose-response relationship such that as stress increased, the likelihood of unhealthy dietary practice also increased'.	Too much 'comfort food' can lead to increased weight, blood pressure and ultimately cardiac problems.
Exercise	Research has indicated that stress may reduce exercise (e.g. Heslop *et al.* 2001; Metcalf *et al.*, 2003) whereas stress management which focuses on increasing exercise has been shown to result in some improvements in coronary health.	Lack of exercise can lead to problems with weight, cardiac fitness and lung function.
Safety	Research suggests that individuals who experience high levels of stress show a greater tendency to perform behaviours that increase their chances of becoming injured (HSE, 2005). Furthermore, some research indicates that the greater the stress, the greater the level of accidents at work and in the car.	Try to focus on the task – otherwise accidents may befall you!

KEY MESSAGE

Coping with stress can lead to more damage if you use inappropriate coping mechanisms.

THINK ABOUT THIS

How does your behaviour change because of stress? How would you suggest you alter your behaviour to cope with the stress?

So, stress can have an influential impact on our health – both physically and mentally. Stress can impact on our physiology, our immune system and the way in which we behave. Consequently, we need to explore how we can minimise stress in both ourselves and our patients. For this we should really explore what variables, or interventions, can be used to try to mediate the stress-poor health link.

QUICK CHECK

List the three routes that can help explain the link between stress and health.

6.7 We need friends - social support

Social support is usually defined as the existence of people on whom we can rely, people who let us know that they care about, value and love us, and the support they provide for us (Sarason *et al.*, 1983). There is a distinction between the existence of social relationships and the functions provided by these. So the structure would be based on 'how many friends, colleagues, family relationships' you have. The functional aspect would refer to what these do.

You can have lots of friends but not interact with them and this may not be very useful – it is better to have one or two close friends rather than lots of distant friends. Social support can come from a variety of different sources and a variety of types of support (Cohen *et al.*, 2000), for example, spouses, relatives, friends, neighbours, co-workers, superiors. But it can also come from professional sources (e.g. the nurse) and this can help reduce stress. The type and amount of social support an individual receives depends upon their social network but also on various demographic factors: their age, sex, culture, socio-economic status and so on.

Generally social support comes in one of five types (see Figure 6.3).

Social support can play an important part in reducing the effects of stress, with the first study suggesting that having close friends can reduce the rates of

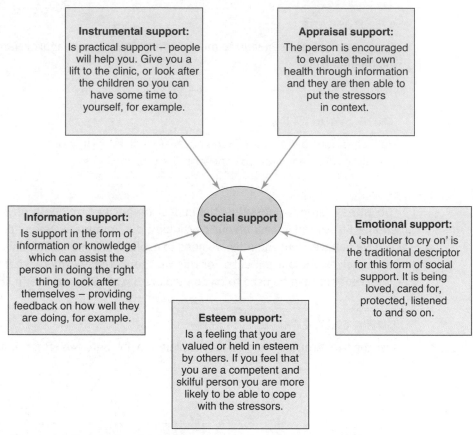

Figure 6.3 **Forms of social support**

mortality (Berkman and Symes, 1979). Subsequent studies have confirmed that reliable links exist between social support and better physical health (e.g. Uchino, 2004). Studies have suggested that those with low levels of social support have higher mortality rates – from cardiovascular disease (e.g. Brummett *et al.*, 2001; Frasure-Smith *et al.*, 2000) or from cancer (e.g. Hibbard and Pope, 1993) and infectious diseases (e.g. Lee and Rotheram-Borus, 2001).

THINK ABOUT THIS

How could you use social support in a nursing setting? Think of a number of examples of how healthcare could be less stressful with the presence of some form of support.

QUICK CHECK

List the five forms of social support.

How does social support protect health?

It has been suggested that social support can protect against the negative effects of stress. There are two main views on why this may be the case.

- **The main effect hypothesis:** social support is beneficial *per se* to health and it is the absence of social support that is stressful. The more social support you have the better because large social networks provide people with regular positive experiences in terms of both emotional as well as physical support. Hence, social support promotes healthier behaviours such as exercise, eating healthily and not smoking, as well as greater adherence to medical regimes.

- **The buffer hypothesis:** social support buffers the individual against the stressor. Rather than protect a person all the time against the minor hassles and stresses of everyday life, the buffer acts when it is needed most. For example, when a person with considerable social support has a diagnosis of an illness then they *appraise* it as less stressful because they know people to whom they can turn. In contrast, those with lower social support might be unable to turn to anyone (Cohen *et al.*, 2000).

Another variable which has been investigated thoroughly is **control** – defined as the extent to which a person feels they are able to change their own circumstances. Broadly, the results suggest that the more control you have in a work situation the less stressful it is. Obviously, there comes a point where you have more control but also considerable responsibility and this can be stressful as well.

QUICK CHECK

What are the models of social support protecting health?

THINK ABOUT THIS

How much control do you have over your current working/study life? Are there any areas over which you would like more control? If you had more control, how do you think it would affect your stress levels?

Stress and hardiness

Kobasa (1979) put forward this concept which describes a set of traits that can protect a person from the effects of stress, and includes control as a factor. A 'hardy' person copes well with stress and is somebody who has a high sense of personal control, is a person who is committed to things and one who likes challenges and sees them as a good thing in life.

Stress and personality

For some people, personality variables are simply a way of behaving. They represent the way a person reacts to stress – their behavioural response. One personality variable that has received much attention is the so-called type A personality type. The definition of a type A behaviour pattern (TABP) is 'an overt pattern of behaviour which is elicited from susceptible individuals in appropriately challenging environment' (Rosenman *et al.*, 1964). TABP was first noted by two US cardiologists (Friedman and Rosenman, 1974) who noted a common type of behaviour in their patients. This behaviour included:

- job involvement;
- excessive hard driving behaviour;
- impatience;
- time urgency;
- competitiveness;
- aggressiveness;
- hostility.

There have been attempts at establishing a link between personality types and other illnesses – most particularly cancer – but these have largely met with limited success (e.g. Dean and Surtees, 1989; Greer *et al.*, 1979; Schapiro *et al.*, 2001).

THINK ABOUT THIS

How would you expect a Type A personality to behave? Think about this in terms of day-to-day activities and when in a healthcare setting.

KEY MESSAGE
Personality variables can influence our physical health.

6.8 How to deal with stress

Given the serious consequences that can arise from stress we will want to try to minimise it as much as possible. Obviously some would argue that in an ideal world, stress would be removed altogether. However, this is unlikely to happen (ever) and, in reality, we don't want this to occur since a small amount of stress is good for us and can lead to enhanced performance in a number of settings.

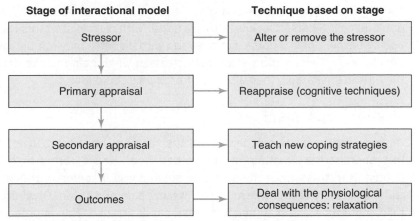

Stage of interactional model	Technique based on stage
Stressor	Alter or remove the stressor
Primary appraisal	Reappraise (cognitive techniques)
Secondary appraisal	Teach new coping strategies
Outcomes	Deal with the physiological consequences: relaxation

Figure 6.4 Stress management techniques based on the interactional model of stress

THINK ABOUT THIS

When is stress a good thing? Is there a good amount, and what happens if it tips over into too much stress?

A number of methods or **stress management techniques** have been devised to try to reduce stress or at least teach people how best to cope with it. Stress management can be defined as the application of methods in psychology to reduce the impact of stress. Each of these methods is based upon the models of stress we discussed earlier, so the link should be simple and clear (see Figure 6.4).

KEY MESSAGE

The model of stress can be used to devise stress management interventions.

QUICK CHECK

List the elements of the interactional model of stress and how a knowledge of this can be used in devising stress management techniques.

Dealing with the stressor

The first method of reducing stress is to remove the stressor, if at all possible! We could take away or modify the demands or exposure to potential stressful conditions. Hence, if the person gets 'stressed out' whenever they ride a horse, don't go near a horse. Obviously, this is easier with certain stressors than others – you can avoid riding a horse, but a person with diabetes may not be able to avoid dealing with needles. If a person gets stressed when going to the dentist and if they avoid the dentist, then all sorts of problems could follow.

Primary appraisal

If the person cannot avoid the stressor then perhaps attempting to get the person to reappraise the situation may prove beneficial. Hence, rather than seeing the dentist as a stressor, get the person to see the visit in a more positive light – this will improve my teeth, my smile, remove my pain and so on. Obviously, this can take some time and may need professional assistance. This approach underlies many cognitive-behavioural interventions and assertiveness training.

Secondary appraisal: improving coping strategies

One of the major psychological approaches to stress management is cognitive-behavioural and this is best developed in the stress-inoculation-training method (Meichenbaum and Cameron, 1983). This is a self-instructional method for teaching individuals to cope with stress and is basically concerned with developing the individual's competence to adapt to stressful events. The individual who is stressed is taught how to cope better – perhaps by being more assertive in a work situation or learning how to cope with the stresses of exams or practice.

Outcomes: dealing with the stress reaction

Finally, stress management can address stress responses directly through **relaxation training**, **biofeedback**, **visual imagery** and **meditation techniques**. The basic premise of relaxation for stress is that it is the opposite of arousal – so relaxing should be a good way to reduce stress. A number of methods have been used to induce relaxation. The most frequently mentioned in psychological terms is **progressive muscle relaxation** (PMR). PMR originated from the work of Jacobson in the 1920s and 1930s. Jacobson (1938) proposed that the main mechanism influencing relaxation lies with the patient's ability to tell the difference between tension and relaxation. PMR involves the successive tensing and relaxing of various muscle groups.

> **Putting theory into practice: visual imagery**
>
> When under stress consider using visual imagery such as that described below. Lie or sit down somewhere quiet, where you are able to relax, and then take yourself through the story, describing it in as much detail as possible to yourself:

Imagine yourself walking along a peaceful old country road . . . The sun is warm on your back. The birds are singing. The air is calm and fragrant. As you walk along your mind naturally wanders to the concerns and worries of the day. Then, you come upon a box by the side of the road and it occurs to you that this box is a perfect place to leave your cares behind while you enjoy this time in the country.

You feel lighter as you progress down the road. Soon, you come across an old gate. The gate creaks as you open it and go through. You find yourself in an overgrown garden. Flowers growing where they have seeded themselves. Vines climbing over a fallen tree. Soft green wild grasses. Shade trees. Breathe deeply, smelling the flowers . . . Listen to the birds and insects . . . Feel the gentle breeze warm against your skin . . . All of your senses are alive and responding in pleasure to the peaceful time and place . . .

And so on . . .

Putting theory into practice: example of a progressive muscle relaxation script

Do try this at home with a willing volunteer. Ask your guinea pig to lie or sit down in a nice quiet room, allow them to settle comfortably and close their eyes if they wish. Legs, ankles and arms should be uncrossed. Now read aloud to them the following:

Let all your muscles feel heavy. And let your whole body just sink into the surface beneath . . . Good. This exercise will guide you through the major muscle groups from your feet to your head, asking you to first tense and then relax those muscles. If you have pain in a particular part of your body today don't tense that area. Instead, just notice any tension that may already be there and let go of it.

Become aware of the muscles in your feet and calves. Pull your toes back up toward your knees. Hold your feet in this position . . . Notice the sensations. Now relax your feet and release the tension. Observe any changes in sensations as you let go of the tension . . . Good.

Now tighten the large muscles of your thighs and buttocks. Hold the muscles tense and as you do be aware of the sensations. And now release these muscles allowing them to feel soft as if they're melting into the surface beneath you . . . That's it.

Now keep tensing and relaxing muscle groups in your abdomen, chest, hands and fingers, face and head.

THINK ABOUT THIS

How could you use some of these stress management programmes in your day-to-day practice?

6.9 Does it work?

Research indicates that stress management programmes can result in reduced stress and generally provide better mental health than having no treatment. Studies have also indicated that PMR can lead to improvements in the following:

- **Hypertension and coronary heart disease:** overall, the evidence (Williams *et al.*, 2003) suggests that: 'structured interventions to reduce stress (stress management, meditation, yoga, cognitive therapies, breathing exercises and biofeedback) have been shown to result in short term reductions in BP'.

- **Immune function:** McGregor and colleagues (2004) explored immune function in women with cancer. They found that a psychological intervention to reduce stress resulted in an improved immune function. This improvement was noted both immediately after the programme and three months later when the group was followed up.

- **Mental health:** the role of stress in the development of mental health issues is considerable. For example, there are suggestions that it is involved in the development of substance misuse problems, depression and anxiety disorders.

QUICK CHECK

List the main methods of stress management – how do they relate back to the interactional model of stress?

6.10 Stress and nursing practice

Chronic workplace stress and the related concept of 'burnout' is a widely recognised phenomenon in healthcare workers. There is a considerable literature base on stress and burnout in both qualified and student nurses. The Nursing Stress Scale (Gray-Toft and Anderson, 1981) has been used extensively to investigate stress and its relationship to clinical areas, job satisfaction and well-being. Nursing provides a series of potential stressors and French *et al.* (2000) have identified nine work-place stressors that might impact on nurses:

- conflict with physicians;
- inadequate preparation;
- problems with peers;
- problems with supervisor;
- discrimination;
- workload;
- uncertainty concerning treatment;
- dealing with death, and dying patients;
- dealing with patients and their families.

The outcomes of stress may be severe. Ultimately, it may lead to psychological and physiological distress, low job satisfaction and burnout. Obviously, some of these sources of stress need to address the working and structural conditions in order to ameliorate any problems.

> **KEY MESSAGE**
> **You need to care for yourself, just as much as you care for your patients.**

6.11 Conclusion

Stress is a major part of all our lives. Its impact can be significant and can harm physical and psychological health through a number of pathways. Medical, and more importantly, psychological interventions can help ameliorate and extinguish stress. This can be of benefit to both the patient/client and the healthcare professional.

6.12 Summary

- **Stress is a difficult concept to define, even though it is a feature of our every-day lives.**
- **Stress can be defined as coming from the inside (GAS), from the outside (life events) and as an interaction between the two (transactional model).**
- **Coping with stress can take one of two broad forms: problem focused or emotion focused.**

- Stress has been implicated in mental health and in certain physical illnesses such as coronary heart disease, cancer and some infectious disorders.

- Stress can influence health through a number of routes: through the immune system and because of changes in behaviour are two of the most investigated.

- There are several mediators of the stress–health link. For example, social support, control, hardiness, personality types and hostility have all been suggested as impacting on the stress–health link.

- Social support can prove effective in promoting health and reducing the consequences of stress.

- Stress management techniques include teaching improved coping techniques, increasing social support and promoting relaxation techniques.

- Workplace stress can lead to considerable problems for both individuals and organisations.

YOUR END POINT

Answer the following questions to assess your knowledge and understanding.

1. Which of the following *is not* true of stress?

    (a) The external environment is a potential stressor.

    (b) The response to the stressor is stress or distress.

    (c) The concept of stress involves biochemical, physiological, behavioural and psychological changes.

    (d) All stress is harmful and damaging.

    (e) All of the above.

2. Alarm, resistance and exhaustion describe three stages represented in which model of stress?

    (a) Life events theory

    (b) Self-regulatory model

    (c) Selye's GAS

    (d) Health belief model

    (e) Protection motivation theory.

3. Social support from others is undoubtedly important for human beings, but it *cannot*:

    (a) buffer the impact of high stress

    (b) stave off loneliness

    (c) compensate for the loss of a marriage partner

    (d) promote better health and longevity

    (e) be treated simply as a number.

4. Which of the following is *not* a good method for dealing with stress?

    (a) regular exercise

    (b) increasing alcohol consumption

    (c) eating less fatty foods

    (d) cutting back on sweets

    (e) seeking out support from friends.

5. When would you expect that your immune system would be weakest?

    (a) during summer holidays

    (b) just after receiving good news

    (c) during exam week

    (d) immune activity would remain the same during all of the above

    (e) at coffee break.

Further reading

Ader, R. and Cohen, N. (1975). Behaviourally conditioned immunosuppression. *Psychosomatic Medicine*, 37(4) pp. 333–340.

Grossman, P., Niemann, L., Schmidt, S. and Walach, H. (2004). Mindfulness-based stress reduction and health benefits: A meta-analysis. *Journal of Psychosomatic Research*, 57, pp. 35–43.

Lazarus, R.S. and Folkman, S. (1984). *Stress, Appraisal and Coping*. New York: Springer.

Sapolsky, R.M. (1994). *Why Zebras Don't Get Ulcers*. New York: Freeman.

Schwarzer, R. and Knoll, N. (2007). Functional roles of social support within the stress and coping process: A theoretical and empirical overview. *International Journal of Psychology*, 42(4) pp. 243–252.

Uchino, B.N., Cacioppo, J.T. and Kiecolt-Glaser, J.K. (1996). The relationship between social support and physiological processes: A review with emphasis on underlying mechanisms and implications for health. *Psychological Bulletin*, 119, pp. 488–533.

Weblinks

http://www.stress.org.uk
Stress Management Society. A resource for individuals wishing to de-stress their lives. The website contains useful tips for stress reduction.

http://www.stress-anxiety-depression.org
Stress, Anxiety and Depression Resource Centre. This site provides information on stress, including the causes of stress and how you can manage the stress in your life. The site also details how stress can lead to anxiety and depression.

http://www.guidetopsychology.com/pmr.htm
Progressive muscle relaxation technique. This site contains a comprehensive explanation of the progressive muscle relaxation technique for stress reduction.

http://www.mbsr.co.uk
Mindfulness based stress reduction technique. The site provides detailed information on the mindfulness stress reduction technique.

https://www.pnirs.org
Psychoneuroimmunology Research Society. This site contains details of the latest research and developments in the field of PNI.

Chapter 7

The psychology of pain

LEARNING OUTCOMES

At the end of this chapter you will be able to:

- Understand the definition of pain
- Appreciate the biopsychosocial nature of pain
- Be able to distinguish between chronic and acute pain
- Be able to identify how to assess pain and what to consider during assessment
- Appreciate the various methods through which pain is managed (medical, behavioural, cognitive and multi-modal methods)
- Be aware of the role of psychology in pain.

YOUR STARTING POINT

Answer the following questions to assess your knowledge and understanding of pain and pain management.

1. Which of the following is a measure for pain assessment?

   (a) Speilberger's
   (b) HAD
   (c) Melzack and Wall
   (d) 16-PF
   (e) All of the above.

2. Which factors are the most important in pain perception?

   (a) biological variables
   (b) psychological variables
   (c) social variables
   (d) none of the above
   (e) (a), (b) and (c).

3. Pain behaviours are:

   (a) behaviours that result from acute pain, but not chronic pain
   (b) obvious when reported by the patient
   (c) behaviours that are a manifestation of pain
   (d) helpful in understanding the physiology of pain
   (e) all of the above.

4. The perception of pain can be influenced by:

   (a) anxiety
   (b) learning
   (c) the meaning of the pain
   (d) all the above
   (e) none of the above.

5. According to the gate controlled theory of pain, which factors close the pain gate?

   (a) depression
   (b) boredom
   (c) low activity levels
   (d) focusing on the pain
   (e) none of the above.

7.1 Introduction

As a keen and conscientious student you are probably reading this book over your morning hot coffee. Being fully engrossed in the text, you reach for your mug and sip your black coffee - it burns your tongue and you don't attempt to sip it again (unless you're a bit odd) until you believe the risk of this pain returning has decreased. This is one example of pain - it is something that is an everyday experience and happens to us all. Of course, many will experience more severe instances of **acute pain** in their lifetime, from tripping and falling or burning on hot coffee, to more long-term pain that may accompany **chronic disorders** such as back pain, arthritis and so on.

It is clear from this example that, although extremely unpleasant, pain can serve a useful survival function, assisting us in identifying and avoiding potentially damaging activities (such as drinking boiling liquids). Similarly, from this we would expect that those who do not have this tool and therefore continue to drink boiling water, walk on broken glass and iron their thumbs would not last long, falling victim to nasty injuries and infections.

Pain then is not just a matter of acute pain as a consequence of injury, it also occurs chronically. For example, over 80 per cent of the population will experience disturbing lower back pain problems at some time during their life, and some 30-40 per cent of the population will have experienced a tension headache in the previous year. Together these figures help explain why pain is one of the most common reasons for people to seek healthcare assistance. Not only does this pain have serious consequences for the individual but it also has an impact on society - the costs in terms of lost employment time, sick pay and benefits, visits to healthcare practitioners and medication are considerable.

With pain being a by-product of many problems leading to hospital attendance and procedures conducted within a hospital setting, the minimising of this pain becomes an important role for all healthcare staff, particularly nurses. As a consequence the role of psychology in pain and how nurses can use this knowledge is of central importance. We will begin this chapter by first looking at what pain is and how to categorise it. Following this, methods of assessing pain will be explored and then how this information has been used to select interventions to manage different types of pain.

KEY MESSAGE
Pain is a useful evolutionary tool that can protect us from harm.

7.2 What is pain?

The term pain encompasses a broad range of experiences, from a bang on the knee as you walk into a piece of furniture, to a paper cut, to the sharp internal pressure of a broken collar bone or a chronic dull ache. The International Association for the Study of Pain (IASP) defines pain as:

'An unpleasant sensory and emotional experience associated with actual or potential tissue damage, or described in terms of such damage' (IASP, 1992).

The literature on pain distinguishes between a number of different forms which are worth outlining here. The most commonly referred to distinction relating to pain is between acute and chronic pain. Acute pain is a short-term pain generally resulting from tissue damage or disease. This pain usually improves throughout the tissue healing process.

QUICK CHECK

Define pain.

Chronic pain is a long-term pain, outliving any original tissue damage. There is no agreement of how long pain must last before it is referred to as chronic. Definitions range from more than six weeks, six months or even 12 months! However, the majority of people agree that pain persisting beyond six months can be labelled chronic. Such pains include arthritis, lower back pain and pain associated with cancer. In chronic pain the link between injury and pain is less clear, suggesting there is more to this pain than mere biology and leaving room for the impact of the person's psychology in pain perception. Psychology has played its primary role in the treatment of chronic pain, although it also has a role in acute pain.

The distinction between acute and chronic pain is a general and simplistic division but can be further sub-divided into:

- **recurrent acute pain** caused by benign conditions that are sometimes intense and sometimes disappear (e.g. migraines);
- **intractable-benign pain** is pain that is persistent and never really goes away (e.g. lower back pain);
- **progressive pain** is that which is both continuous and worsens over time (e.g. arthritis or cancer).

QUICK CHECK

What are the various forms of pain?

Another distinction that can be made is between pain's various known or assumed biological causes. There are two groups of pain and these are identified in the following box.

Types of pain, defined by cause (or assumed causes)

Nociceptive (pain resulting from the stimulation of specific pain receptors)
- **Somatic:** pain occurring from stimulation of receptors within tissues such as skin, muscle, joints, bones, and ligaments; often known as musculo-skeletal pain.

- **Visceral:** pain occurring from stimulation of receptors within internal organs of the main body cavities. This pain originates from ongoing injury to the internal organs or the tissues that support them.

Non-nociceptive (pain arising from within the peripheral and central nervous system – assumed to be independent of any initial injury/damage)
- **Neuropathic:** pain occurring from within the nervous system itself – also known as pinched nerve or trapped nerve. The pain may originate from the peripheral nervous system or from the central nervous system. It can result from diseases that affect nerves (such as diabetes), from trauma or because chemotherapy drugs can affect nerves as a consequence of cancer treatment.

- **Sympathetic:** pain that occurs due to possible over-activity of the **sympathetic nervous system** and central/peripheral nervous system mechanisms.

By distinguishing between types of pain the nurse can identify its likely duration and the patient's response to possible pain treatments.

THINK ABOUT THIS

What sort of pain have you experienced in your life? What memories do you have of being in pain? How were they different from each other? Can you categorise them into different forms? How did you treat the different forms of pain?

With these distinctions in mind it is important to realise that a biological cause for pain is not always present and that psychological factors have an important role to play in all aspects of pain. As pain is not experienced independently from our culture or social situation, or our upbringing (e.g. what we have learnt about injury, how our friends see us, whether the expression of pain is appropriate), then we have to appreciate that:

> 'Psychological factors are always present, whether or not they are acknowledged by patients or therapists. They can be ignored, although their effect on pain may be powerful, or they can be systematically managed in such a way as to maximise pain relief' (IASP, 1992).

QUICK CHECK

What are the biopsychosocial elements of pain?

THINK ABOUT THIS

Think back to your experiences of pain. What social, individual, cultural or biological factors may have influenced how it was perceived? Can you classify them into biological, psychological or social factors? List them under the following headings:

BIO   **PSYCHO**   **SOCIAL**

KEY MESSAGE

Pain is a biopsychosocial concept.

7.3 Concepts of pain

Attempts at understanding pain have a long history, with one of the first explanations being provided by Descartes in 1644 who:

> 'Conceived of the pain system as a straight through channel from the skin to the brain' (Melzack and Wall, 1973:126).

In other words, when you hit your thumb with a hammer the hurt and damage from this area is sent up to the brain via one channel that tells you that you are experiencing pain.

A development of this theory was the **specificity theory** developed by Von Frey in 1894 who assumed that there were specific sensory receptors responsible for the transmission of sensation, warmth and pain. In a similar discussion,

Goldschneider (1920) developed the pattern theory of pain which suggested that the pattern of nerve impulses determined the degree of pain and that messages from the damaged area were sent to the brain via these nerve impulses.

These are rather simple ways of viewing the pain process, all of which have the same series of underlying principles:

- damage to the body causes the sensation of pain;
- psychological reactions are a consequence of the pain;
- no psychological variables are associated with modifying the pain;
- pain is an automatic response;
- pain has a single cause;
- there are only two forms of pain – organic ('real' pain when an injury is visible) or psychogenic ('all in the patient's mind').

If we were to visualise this process it might look something like this:

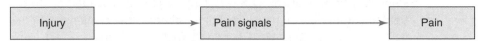

If these models were correct then it should be relatively easy to treat pain by interfering with activity in pain pathways:

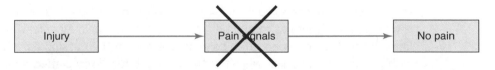

This model of pain (known as the **linear-biomedical model**) is still around today and underlies surgical treatments discussed later in this chapter.

> **THINK ABOUT THIS**
>
> What evidence are you aware of that might bring a simple link between injury and pain into question? What do you do when you experience pain in an attempt to reduce it? Why do these activities/behaviours work?

> **QUICK CHECK**
>
> What is the linear-biomedical model of pain?

Problems with earlier models

This earlier view of pain as a simple linear concept was very popular up until the 20th century when evidence to suggest that pain was not as simple as a mere linear relationship between injury and perceived pain started to mount up. So what evidence do we have against this view of pain?

Firstly, it was noted that when attempts were made to interfere with these pain signals through biological interventions such as medication or surgery, the treatment was not as useful for more persistent or chronic pain.

Secondly, it was observed that two people reporting the same level of injury in the same location did not necessarily report the same level of pain and often required differing levels of pain relief. This suggested that pain was not simply a direct response to a given stimulus. A classic study which reported on this phenomenon is that of Beecher (1959). He reported on the pain experiences of civilians compared to soldiers returning from the battlefield). He found that similar levels of tissue damage needed greater levels of pain medication in the civilian group compared to soldiers. Only one in three soldiers required pain killers, whereas in the civilian group it was four out of five. Beecher suggested that it was the meaning of the situation that was affecting the pain experience. The soldiers' pain was offset by the fact that they had escaped death on the battlefield and were now on their way home, whereas the civilians' pain had singularly negative connotations. This suggests that pain in itself is not simply a consequence of excited nerve impulses, but that psychological and social factors play a part.

Another form of evidence is that of **phantom limbs** where there are no nerve transmissions but there is pain: in other words the part of the body where the pain is reported isn't there so cannot be responsible for the pain. People who have lost limbs through amputation often have severe pain in the missing limbs. Phantom limb pain has no physical basis but the pain can feel excruciating and as if it is spreading. Not only is the pain not related to actual tissue damage but not all people who have had a limb amputated experience this pain, or the level of pain may vary from individual to individual.

These pieces of evidence – the variation in medication's success at reducing pain, the variation in people's perception of pain relating to the same tissue damage and pain without injury – indicate the pain process to be more complex than the linear-biomedical model, and that pain does not equate to injury.

7.4 The gate control theory of pain

In order to overcome some of these identified problems, Melzack (a psychologist) and Wall (an anatomist) published a new theory of pain: **the gate control theory** (Melzack and Wall, 1965). It described a role for both physiological causes and interventions and psychological causes and interventions. The simple description of the gate control theory is that pain is a consequence of pain messages. However, importantly, these pain messages travel through a gate – if the gate is open then more pain messages get through and hence more pain is experienced (see

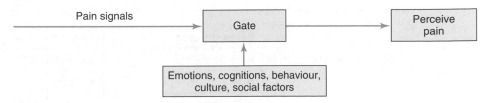

Figure 7.1 The gate control theory of pain

Figure 7.1). On the other hand, if the gate is closed then fewer pain messages get through and so less pain is experienced.

The central idea of the gate control theory is the presence of neural mechanisms in the spinal cord which can somehow close or open a gate, and so alter the amount of pain messages travelling to the brain. The theory proposes that the gating mechanism is in the **substantia gelatinosa** of the **dorsal horns**, which are part of the **grey matter** of the spinal cord.

> **QUICK CHECK**
>
> What is the gate control theory of pain?

In the model you can see that signals from the injury enter the gating mechanism (substantia gelatinosa) of the spinal cord from pain fibres (**A-delta** and **C fibres**). After these signals pass through the gating mechanism they activate transmission cells which send impulses to the brain. When the signals reach a critical level the person perceives pain: the greater the output beyond this level, the greater the pain intensity. When the pain signals enter the spinal cord and the gate is open the transmission cells send impulses freely. But if the gate is closed then the output of the transmission cells is inhibited. This leads us to the big question, what open or closes the gate?

● The amount of activity in the pain fibre: the greater the injury the more active the pain fibres, the more open the gate, meaning larger injuries often cause more pain than smaller ones.

● The amount of activity in other peripheral fibres: some small fibres, A-beta fibres, carry information about harmless stimuli (e.g. touching or rubbing of the skin) and tend to close the gate. Hence, you can rub a cut better.

● Messages that descend from the brain: impulses from **neurons** in the brainstem and **cortex** can open or close the gate. The effects of some of these (e.g. anxiety or excitement) may open or close the gate, so what would normally bring a child to tears goes unnoticed when they are having fun with their friends at their birthday party.

Other factors in the negotiation of pain signals are presented in Table 7.1. Many of these factors may be visible in your own and others' natural responses to pain (e.g. rubbing it better).

Table 7.1 Factors influencing pain

	Opens the gate	Closes the gate
Emotional factors	● Anxiety	● Happiness
	● Worry	● Optimism
	● Tension	● Relaxation
	● Depression	
Cognitive and behavioural factors	● Focusing on the pain	● More involvement and interest in life activities
	● Boredom	● Distractions or focus on other activities
	● Other reactions	● Other reactions
Physical factors	● Extent and type of injury	● Medication
	● Low activity level	● Counter-stimulation (e.g. rubbing)

THINK ABOUT THIS

How could you use these ideas to develop an intervention for managing pain without medical treatment?

KEY MESSAGE

The gate control theory suggests that a variety of physiological, psychological or social factors can open (i.e. make pain worse) or close (i.e. relieve pain) the gate and hence alter the perception of pain.

QUICK CHECK

What can open and close the gate?

Problems with the gate control theory

Obviously the gate control theory considers a number of aspects not addressed by a more linear biological model and consequently has advanced our understanding of pain. The model has also stimulated a wealth of additional pain research. Most, although not all, of these studies have offered support for the proposals. Nevertheless there are still several problems with the model that have been highlighted:

- Although a great deal of investigation has centred on the search for the neural mechanism of the 'gate' there has been little advance in locating this mechanism.
- The model still focuses on physiological rather than psychological input: an organic basis for the factors impacting on pain is still assumed (it is not the emotion but the chemical basis of the emotion that is relevant).
- Although the gate control theory attempts to integrate mind and body it still sees them as separate processes.

However, this being said, the gate control theory has moved the concept forward considerably from the original linear-biomedical approach.

7.5 Psychological factors influencing pain

On the back of the development of the gate control theory considerable research has explored the psychosocial factors of pain. This research has indicated that there are many factors that can influence pain. For example, **self-efficacy** – the extent to which somebody believes they are able to cope with pain – can influence their pain perception (Rahman *et al.*, 2008). Similarly, the way in which a person copes with challenges (e.g. an **emotion-focused** vs. **problem-focused approach**) can influence their success in managing pain experiences (Elfant *et al.*, 2008).

KEY MESSAGE

If a person believes they have control over their own pain they will experience less of it.

This research supports the need to look at pain in terms of individual experience and consider the factors important in each person's case. As you can see from what has been discussed so far, attempting to measure pain objectively will be difficult. Nevertheless, it is essential in the treatment of pain to understand the nature of the pain experienced; this can help practitioners distinguish between the types of pain and for them to focus on the evidence base relating to the management of this type of pain. We will now consider some of the methods used to assess the total pain experience.

7.6 The assessment of pain

In order to assess pain it is important to understand the way the *individual* patient experiences it and to ensure that all of the components of the pain experience are assessed. Consequently, most measures of pain include at least three dimensions:

● sensory: the nature, location and intensity of pain;

● affective: the emotional component and response to the pain;

● impact: functioning, level of activity and participation in daily life.

On this basis we can evaluate the individual's readiness for treatment and develop an appropriate intervention which focuses on the specific pain experience of each patient. We can also monitor the effectiveness of any intervention applied to the pain and modify treatment based on these findings.

There are a number of issues that will influence how a nurse should measure pain. Why, who and for how long you want to review will all influence this selection process. Let's now look at some of the options available.

QUICK CHECK

What are the elements of pain measurement?

THINK ABOUT THIS

When you are in pain, what sorts of components does this have? How would you assess the pain (e.g. location, duration and so on)?

Self-report measures

The most obvious thing to do when you want to know about somebody else's experience is to ask them about it. There are a number of methods for approaching this: from the **unstructured interview** to the more formally structured **rating scale**. Interview discussions can focus on such items as the history of the pain, where the pain is, what it feels like and when it tends to occur, how strong it is, what treatments have been tried and what have/have not worked, emotional adjustment and the social context of the pain. In any format, the gathering of a detailed pain history is vital in understanding the patient's pain experience and the possible causes or factors involved in this experience.

There are four categories of pain assessment tool which are reported that provide a useful guiding framework:

● uni-dimensional

● numerical

- categorical
- multidimensional.

Uni-dimensional measures

Uni-dimensional tools record a single aspect of the pain (e.g. the degree of pain relief or pain intensity). This is then compared throughout the treatment processes. The advantage of the pain relief scale is that comparisons can be made between interventions, as all participants start with a baseline of zero. However, this type of measurement does not take into account the complexity of the pain experience and as such will not give a full picture of the impact of treatments on the pain experience.

Numerical measures

Numerical assessments such as the **visual analogue scale** (VAS) involve patients rating their pain on a scale of 0–10; 0 indicating no pain and 10 the most extreme pain (see Figure 7.2). This may be represented as a list of numbers or as a 10 mm line on which patients mark their current position.

These scales have the advantage of being quick and simple to administer, but although categorised as separate to that of uni-dimensional measures, these too can assess only one aspect of the pain experience.

Categorical measures

A variation on the VAS is the **verbal rating scale** (VRS) where people are asked to describe their pain by choosing a word or phrase from several that are given (see, for example, Figure 7.3). These scales can be used to measure how someone estimates

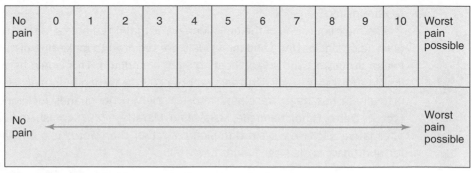

Figure 7.2 Example of a numerical measure of pain

No pain	Some pain	Considerable pain	Worst pain possible

Figure 7.3 Example of a verbal rating scale

their pain in general and how this changes over time, either with or without treatment. Again this approach is quick and easy to administer, but improvements in the pain experience are more difficult to identify when comparing these responses than numerical scores. Adjustment from one category to another may require a greater degree of improvement than does a 5 mm shift along a line.

Multidimensional measures

The self-report measures discussed so far only inform us of one element of an overall experience. Healthcare professionals are now recognising the multidimensional nature of pain, which suggests that these scales may be too simplistic to cover the full nature of the pain process. Melzack (1975) developed the **McGill pain questionnaire** (MPQ), one of the first widely used multidimensional pain assessment measures developed based on observations and some intensive research.

The McGill pain questionnaire focuses on location, quality, intensity and sensory dimensions of pain. The measurement tool first uses a verbal descriptive scale consists of 102 pain descriptors which are sorted into groups describing different aspects of pain. These are classified into three major groups of words (e.g. sensory, quivering, pulsing; affective, punishing, growling; evaluative, annoying, troublesome). People in acute pain tend to score higher on the sensory descriptors while those in chronic pain score more highly on the emotional words. It has also been noted that people suffering from the same sort of conditions choose the same pattern of words. In addition the questionnaire investigates the pain location, medication and previous pain, change in pain over time (e.g. what things may have increased or relieved it) and a verbal rating scale of present pain intensity (PPI). There is also a short form of this questionnaire available which includes 15 descriptive words and takes only a couple of minutes to administer.

The main limitation of the questionnaire is that it requires a fairly strong vocabulary (e.g. 'lancinating') and individuals are required to make fine distinctions between groups of words (e.g. 'beating' and 'pounding'). This would be particularly limiting for those reporting their experience in a second language. However, the instrument has been translated into a variety of languages including German, French, Dutch, Hindi, Kannada, Malayalam, Marathi, Urdu, Spanish and Chinese. An alternative is to use a scale with pictures rather than words (e.g. the Wong-Baker facial grimace scale – see Figure 7.4).

Physiological measures

Although there are no objective measures of pain, physiological measures may be used to assess associated factors such as heart rate. These measures include, for example, **electromyography** (EMG) – see Figure 7.5 – which can be used to

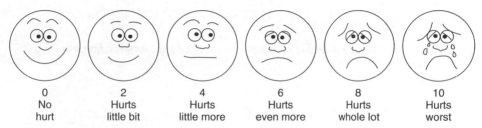

0	2	4	6	8	10
No hurt	Hurts little bit	Hurts little more	Hurts even more	Hurts whole lot	Hurts worst

Figure 7.4 The Wong-Baker Faces Pain Rating Scale

Source: From Hockenberry M. J., Wilson, D. *Wong's Essentials of Paediatric Nursing* edn 8, St Louis, 2009, Mosby. Used with permission. Copyright Mosby.

QUICK CHECK

With what population would you use the Wong-Baker facial grimace scale?

measure muscle tension in patients with headaches and lower-back pain. This approach not only investigates a possible cause of pain but also indicates a possible method of intervention (see progressive muscle relaxation later in the chapter). However, most research using these measures has failed to demonstrate a consistent relationship between these physiological measures and the experience of pain as obviously a number of other factors can affect these results.

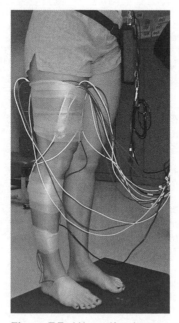

Figure 7.5 Attempting to measure pain with an EMG

Behavioural measures

Another factor influenced by pain is outward behaviour. These are behavioural measures which assess the behaviours associated with pain, either by counting them or observing how they change over time: for example, physical symptoms (e.g. limping or rubbing), verbal expressions (e.g. groaning or sighing) or facial expressions (e.g. grimacing or frowning). These measures are generally useful and can be used either in everyday situations or in structured clinical sessions. These observations may be used in addition to information gained from self-reports. One limitation of this approach is that it may be more difficult to apply to the assessment of chronic or recurrent pain because the overt behavioural signs usually associated with pain tend to become habit as time passes, making them difficult to observe reliably in those with chronic pain. These behaviours are also easily faked or modified based on what patients perceive is expected of them.

A non-verbal measure of pain is the checklist of nonverbal pain indicators (CNPI) developed by Feldt (2000) which can be used in a range of different settings – see Table 7.2.

Table 7.2 Checklist of nonverbal pain indicators (CNPI)

Behaviour	With movement	At rest
1. Vocal complaints: nonverbal (sighs, gasps, moans, groans, cries)		
2. Facial grimaces/winces (furrowed brow, narrowed eyes, clenched teeth, tightened lips, jaw drop, distorted expressions)		
3. Bracing (clutching or holding onto furniture, equipment or affected area during movement)		
4. Restlessness (constant or intermittent shifting of position, rocking, intermittent or constant hand motions, inability to keep still)		
5. Rubbing (massaging affected area)		
6. Vocal complaints: verbal (words expressing discomfort or pain – 'ouch', 'that hurts'; cursing during movement; exclamations of protest – 'stop', 'that's enough')		

Scoring

Score a 0 if the behaviour was not observed. Score a 1 if the behaviour occurred even briefly during activity or at rest. The total number of indicators is summed for the behaviours observed at rest, with movement, and overall. There are no clear cutoff scores to indicate severity of pain; instead, the presence of any of the behaviours may be indicative of pain, warranting further investigation, treatment and monitoring by the practitioner.

THINK ABOUT THIS

In what types of situation and with which types of patient would you use the CNPI?

QUICK CHECK

What sort of behaviours are associated with pain? How can you assess these?

Assessing children's pain

As you can see, some of these measures rely heavily on verbal communication (with the exception of the CNPI), so obviously assessing the pain of an articulate adult would involve different measures to those we would expect to be applied to a child. Therefore these methods need to be adapted to the individual patient; for example, pre-verbal children have to be assessed through observational methods (e.g. facial expressions, crying) while older children can be assessed through picture-based pain scales (e.g. the picture scale (Frank *et al.*, 1982)).

Assessing the pain of older people

Similarly, assessing older patients introduces other issues. Older people are often reluctant to acknowledge or report pain and the increase in such problems as sensory impairment and memory loss at this age can make communicating effectively with this group equally difficult (Royal College of Physicians, British Geriatrics Society, British Pain Society, 2007).

When using self-reports or interviewing patients from these groups it may also be beneficial to consult with others close to the patient, such as family members or carers, in order to expand the level and breadth of information available to you.

The FLACC scale

The Faces, Legs, Activity, Cry, Consolability (FLACC) Scale relies on behavioural indicators to assess pain. This multidimensional tool is a checklist that guides the healthcare professional in examining the child's behaviour in response to pain. This checklist was developed for children aged two to seven years for use after surgery or when experiencing sharp, acute pain during a procedure.

Face

0	1	2
No particular expression or smile	Occasional grimace or frown, withdrawn, disinterested	Frequent to constant frown, clenched jaw, quivering chin

Legs

0	1	2
Normal position or relaxed	Uneasy, restless, tense	Kicking or legs drawn up

Activity

0	1	2
Lying quietly, normal position, moves easily	Squirming, shifting back/forth, tense	Arched, rigid or jerking

Cry

0	1	2
No cry, awake or asleep	Moans or whimpers, occasional complaint	Crying steadily, screams or sobs, frequent complaints

Consolability

0	1	2
Content, relaxed	Reassured by occasional touching, hugging, or 'talking to', distractible	Difficult to console or comfort

How to use the FLACC scale:

● Rate the patient on each of the five categories (i.e. Face, Legs, Arms, Cry, Consolability). Each category is scored on the 0–2 scale.

- Add the scores together (for a total possible score of 0-10).
- Document the total pain score.

Interpreting the score:
  0 = Relaxed and comfortable
 1-3 = Mild discomfort
 4-6 = Moderate pain
 7-10 = Severe pain or discomfort or both

THINK ABOUT THIS

How would you assess pain in these cases:

- a 6-month-old child undergoing orthopaedic treatment;
- a 27-year-old man with paranoid schizophrenia with a cut forehead;
- a 33-year-old woman with chronic lower back pain;
- an 18-year-old woman undergoing dental treatment;
- an 88-year-old adult with dementia following a fall;
- a 16-year-old man with learning disabilities complaining of stomach pain?

KEY MESSAGE

There are different forms of pain assessment, dependent on the population, the nature of the pain and the injury.

7.7 The management of pain

It is very often the case that the elimination of pain is not a realistic goal, therefore it is more common to refer to the management of pain, in which interventions are aimed at improving the situation of the patient without the intention of removing pain altogether (although this would obviously be ideal!). This terminology also affects the way in which patients perceive, and what they expect from, the treatment. Expecting pain to be eliminated altogether may be an unrealistic goal which could lead to negative impacts on the individual's quality of life and overall mental health.

The management of different types of pain, particularly acute pain and chronic pain, is obviously different. You are unlikely to give someone with a severe leg injury a single aspirin and expect it to relieve their pain, although this may be sufficient for a mild headache. Nevertheless, there are common elements in the form of approaches that may be useful for different types of pain: for example it is likely that someone who has a severe leg injury is likely to be offered some form of **medication intervention**. It may also be that those with chronic pain benefit from some form of psychological support and intervention as this may be useful in managing their pain.

In this section each of these types of approaches will be explored and their application to both acute and chronic pain will be discussed. The benefits and problems for the nurse and patient for each of these approaches will also be outlined. However, with all of these approaches it is important to remember that there is no single answer to pain; if this were the case you would expect this section to be considerable shorter, but in actual fact **multi-modal methods** are often required.

> ### KEY MESSAGE
> Pain management requires more than just medical means.

Methods of pain management

The most obvious method of pain management is by medication intervention which temporarily reduces/relieves pain but does not eliminate its cause. These are most useful in reducing acute pain and can be extremely effective. There are many forms of drugs that can be taken to reduce acute pain and three of the most common are listed in Table 7.3.

Although effective drug treatments are available, not all patients receive appropriate pain relief 'resulting in the needless suffering of countless millions of patients' (IASP, 1992: 3). This is in part the result of pain medication being administered based on what health professionals expect to be the problem as opposed to resulting from a consultation with the patient about the nature of their pain experience. This may result in many patients remaining in pain. A survey of over 3000 individuals discharged from hospital showed that some 87 per cent reported moderate or severe pain on leaving hospital (Bruster *et al.*, 1994). In children the picture is the same: Karling *et al.* (2002) reported that almost

Table 7.3 **Methods of drug pain management**

Pain-analgesic	How it works
Aspirin and ibuprofen	Reduces fever and inflammation by interfering with the transmission of pain signals.
Narcotics (e.g. codeine and morphine)	Inhibits the transmission of pain signals and can be very effective at reducing severe pain.
Local anaesthetics (e.g. for tooth pain or for an epidural)	Blocks the nerve cells in a small region from generating impulses.

three-quarters of those children discharged were in pain and that a quarter of these were experiencing moderate or severe pain. This, coupled with the length of hospital stays reducing, means that the need for effective pain management at home is essential.

As indicated in the Beecher (1959) study, people often respond differently to pain and this can affect the treatment offered and requested. A difference in response to pain by different ethnic groups has been identified, with different groups expressing the quality and intensity or frequency of pain differently and using varying amounts of analgesics in an attempt to control their pain, which illustrates the influence of culture on pain perception (Cleland *et al.*, 2005). The prescribing of pain medication may also be influenced by the healthcare professional's expectations of the patient. For example, it is suggested that men are viewed as 'tough' or 'macho' and hence are often prescribed less medication than a woman irrespective of the individual's rating of pain.

KEY MESSAGE

Drug management of pain must be optimal.

QUICK CHECK

Highlight three methods of medical pain management. What types of pain can they be used for?

Surgical methods

Another intervention resulting from the **medical model** of treatment is the surgical approach. Obviously mild headaches would not be best tackled through surgery; on the other hand, this intervention may be considered if the pain becomes severe or persistents.

As mentioned when looking at concepts of pain, the thinking behind surgical approaches to pain management/reduction is relatively simple: if the pain pathway to the brain is broken then the pain message cannot get through. Hence surgery involves the division of nerve pathways, either by severing or destroying them, thus reducing the perception of pain. This technique is most commonly used in those with chronic lower-back pain (mainly in the USA).

However, as predicted from evidence refuting this simple linear link, the technique is not particularly successful and there may be limited benefits. Indeed, there may be some negative consequences resulting from the removal of these pathways: numbness, pins and needles and even paralysis in the region involved in the surgery. Furthermore, since pain messages can travel to the brain via different routes the pain may return a month or two after the surgery.

THINK ABOUT THIS

In what circumstances would surgical treatment of pain be appropriate?

Transcutaneous electrical nerve stimulation (TENS)

A further method of interfering with the pain signals is through the use of **transcutaneous electrical nerve stimulation** (TENS). This works on the premise of replacing pain signals with a tingling sensation through the stimulation of the skin area over the site of the pain, using an electrical stimulator. This is similar to when you rub your knee after banging it: stimulation of the receptors around the pain site can reduce the overall perception of pain. This form of pain management is reported to be effective for some individuals in some forms of chronic conditions: phantom limb pain, labour and pain following surgery. However, despite being extensively used there is conflicting evidence about whether TENS is beneficial (Khadilkar *et al.*, 2008). The major methodological problem has been the lack of sufficient numbers and placebo-control groups in the studies, a trend you will see throughout research on the value of pain management techniques.

KEY MESSAGE

TENS machines can be useful as a pain management tool, particularly in labour.

Biofeedback

Another approach used to manage pain through the modifying of biological processes is **biofeedback**. This technique involves the monitoring of physiological data (e.g. heart rate, muscle activity, brain wave patterns and skin response) which is then presented to the patient who attempts to control and change these originally involuntary biological variables. For example, a patient's muscle group is wired to an electromyography (EMG) machine and the results of the muscle tension presented to the patient. The patient is then shown how the muscle tension can be increased or decreased – by either tensing their muscles or relaxing. By providing feedback on how the biological variables respond, the patient over time learns how to control their physiological responses by changing thoughts or behaviour.

Biofeedback has been used in cases such as tension headaches, migraines and lower back pain. Vasudeva *et al.* (2003) reported that using biofeedback techniques in those with migraine headaches reduced their reports of pain, depression and anxiety. The biofeedback treatment involved the patients learning to control their cerebral blood flow velocity which was measured in the middle **cerebral artery** with a **transcranial doppler**. However, biofeedback can often be time consuming and expensive, especially as it is often considered nothing more than relaxation.

Relaxation

Relaxation is most commonly used as a treatment for tension headaches or migraines (see also Chapter 6). The thinking behind these relaxation approaches to tension headaches, for example, is relatively straightforward: tension headaches are assumed to result from persistent muscle contractions around the head, neck and shoulders and if this occurs then relaxing these muscles should have the opposite effect: the person becomes relaxed and pain free (there are, of course, other theories of headache development).

Since there appears to be a link between the tension and the pain then a suitable intervention would be **progressive muscle relaxation** (PMR). In essence the PMR approach involves the tensing and relaxing of muscles to demonstrate to the patient the difference between the two. The patient is then taught how best to relax. They will also be taught to identify the signs of an onset of a pain episode so they can start to relax early to prevent the pain from increasing. It is not only the PMR method that can be used to relax and reduce the tension and hence the pain, there are a number of other forms of relaxation techniques.

Research into the issue of whether relaxation works for a range of pains has produced mixed results (e.g. Sarafino and Goehring, 2000), with most research reviewed in the literature displaying weaknesses in methodology, which limit the ability to draw conclusions about this intervention. Relaxation appears to benefit some but not others and as it has little if any negative impact on patients it is generally agreed that relaxation should be integrated into approaches to reduce pain as part of a multi-modal intervention. Whether relaxation is effective as a standalone intervention is debatable.

With this in mind it must be noted that the encouragement to 'take it easy' and to avoid social, leisure and work activities is not classed as a relaxation technique as such and may lead to negative impacts. Reductions in these activities can lead to patients becoming more and more inactive over and beyond the recommended rest period. Ultimately, they may avoid more activities and this can cause an increased focus on the pain since they no longer have any other outlets on which to focus. Their lives tend to revolve around the pain and its treatment. As a loss of rewards from the environment continues there is an increase in depression. Finally depression can lead to a greater increase in pain and a vicious downward spiral can develop.

THINK ABOUT THIS

In what situations would relaxation be useful as a method of pain management?

QUICK CHECK

Using the material throughout this book, think of a relaxation strategy for pain management.

Acupuncture

Acupuncture is aimed at channelling the body's motivational energy in an effort to stimulate the body's natural healing response and to restore balance. Developed in the Far East, this method is now being used more and more as a complementary therapy to tackle pain. Reviews suggest that there is evidence both for and against the effectiveness of this treatment (Furlan *et al.*, 2005).

There are a range of approaches to acupuncture and a variety of **control methods** have been used to evaluate its effectiveness: these variations make an examination of acupuncture's value as a pain intervention difficult to assess. Therefore, clinical research into the use of acupuncture as an effective treatment is currently difficult to interpret (Birch *et al.*, 2004).

Hypnotism

Hypnosis refers to an altered state of consciousness brought about by a trained therapist. There are anecdotal reports of hypnotised patients undergoing cardiac surgery, caesarean sections and appendectomies with no medication. There are two main schools of thought about the effectiveness of hypnosis in the treatment of chronic pain: it works (e.g. Barber, 1998) or it works merely as a placebo or as a relaxation technique (e.g. Spanos and Katsanis, 1989). Overall, however, the evidence is not substantial enough to be used in place of psychological or medical methods in the treatment of pain.

Recent developments with the use of hypnosis in children have explored the role of virtual reality in this process and introduced a range of new possibilities (Patterson *et al.*, 2006).

THINK ABOUT THIS

How would you manage pain in these cases (using both medical and psychological approaches):

- a 6-month-old child undergoing orthopaedic treatment;
- a 27-year-old man with paranoid schizophrenia with a cut forehead;
- a 33-year-old woman with chronic lower back pain;
- an 18-year-old woman undergoing dental treatment;
- an 88-year-old adult with dementia following a fall;
- a 16-year-old man with learning disabilities complaining of stomach pain?

7.8 Behavioural approaches to pain and pain management

Behavioural approaches (see Chapter 2 for more details) to the treatment of pain argue that pain is a series of pain behaviours (or **operants**) and that pain can either be increased by reinforcing these pain behaviours (i.e. **positive reinforcement**) or decreased by individuals avoiding an unpleasant or aversive situation (i.e. **negative reinforcement**). For example, it is argued that people in pain often receive certain benefits and that this may reinforce their behaviour: if an individual loses their stressful job but receives compensation they will avoid the stress and burden associated with a stressful job as well as benefiting from the compensation. There might be other benefits as well – others within the family may fulfil the domestic chores and so these pressures will be removed (negative reinforcement). In addition, they may receive the sympathy and attention of friends and family and have more spare time to engage in other activities (positive reinforcement).

KEY MESSAGE

Pain behaviours can be rewarded by well-meaning family and friends of the patient.

This approach was first applied by Fordyce *et al.* (1984). In a behavioural approach the pain behaviours are noted: for example, how often the patient makes an audible remark (e.g. moaning), expression (e.g. grimacing teeth), distorted posture or movement (e.g. limping), negative affect (e.g. depression) or avoidance of activity (e.g. not walking). The behavioural approach deals with these behaviours. Initially the patient is asked to do something small (e.g. walk a few paces) and this is reinforced by the healthcare practitioners and the family. In contrast to negative reinforcement, the pain behaviours are left unrewarded. Hence, the grimaces are ignored and not reinforced by healthcare professionals. At the same time the pain medication is reduced and given on a time-based schedule rather than on need as expressed by the patient. Over time this period is lengthened and/or the dosage reduced. This environment allows for more positive behaviours to be reinforced

THINK ABOUT THIS

Think about a recent case of somebody in pain you have come across in your practice. How would you assess pain behaviours? What sort of pain behaviours did the patient show? How were these behaviours being reinforced? What sort of difficulties do you think you would face when attempting to alter these behaviours?

and pain behaviours to be extinguished. Important to the behavioural approach is the patient's family. It has been found that those with chronic pain are more likely to have 'caring' and 'over-supportive' families. Hence the patient's family are trained not to reinforce pain behaviours by not providing sympathy or taking on more of the domestic work.

These interventions have been shown to be successful in reducing their target pain behaviours, resulting in reduced use of pain medication, increased activity levels and so on (Roelofs et al., 2002), particularly when family and friends are supporting this approach. Therefore the behavioural functioning of patients can be improved through these techniques. Nevertheless, as these activities are not a direct objective measure of pain, their reduction cannot automatically be assumed to be associated with reduced pain.

Indeed, Roelofs et al. (2002) also suggest that there is evidence that there is no reduction in subjective measures of pain. Overall, therefore, patients may still re-port the same amount of pain, but not show it. Furthermore, detractors of the be-havioural approach argue that as soon as the intervention ends the old pattern of inactivity and pain behaviour reappears. It should also be evident that this type of programme may not be suitable for all – certainly those with progressive chronic pain (e.g. cancer sufferers) would not benefit in the long term. In addition to this, although these types of approaches can be effective in the long term they can be hard for the patient to complete and there is a large drop-out rate from pro-grammes with this form of intervention. In certain cases this drop-out rate can be as much as one-third of all participants.

Finally, reviews suggest that many of the behavioural trials in the current liter-ature should perhaps be construed as behavioural plus medication treatments, or behavioural treatment following non-optimal medication treatment, as few stud-ies have systematically isolated pure behavioural treatments (Andrasik, 2007).

KEY MESSAGE

It is not always beneficial to the patient's pain management to be supportive and remove them from their usual practices and routines.

QUICK CHECK

What are refinforcers and how can pain behaviours be reinforced?

7.9 Cognitive approaches

Instead of the focus on outward pain behaviour, cognitive therapists, as the name would suggest, stress that the way people think is important in their experience of pain. It is these thoughts that are the target for change in any cognitive programme.

If we take the example of someone who is waiting in the reception area for a dentist appointment, a number of thoughts maybe going through this person's head: 'this is going to hurt', 'I don't want them to use those drills', 'I am really anxious'. These thoughts are likely to increase the pain experienced. Research by Ulrich (2006) lends support for the idea that those with high anxiety amplify pain anticipation which influences their evaluation of treatment-related pain. Similarly research into pain perceived to be intentional and that which is non-intentional lends further support to the role of cognitions in pain perception, with those believing the behaviour leading to pain to have been intentional experiencing a higher level of pain than those who believed it to be an accident (Lavoie, 2008).

If we return to the dentist situation and reverse these **cognitions**, someone may be waiting and thinking 'I am going to be brave . . . there are experiences a lot more painful than this . . . it won't take long', this is more likely to reduce tension and the experience of pain. This is known as **reconceptualisation,** viewing the same experience in a more positive light to elicit different beliefs about the event.

You can use three elements of cognitive therapy with your patients:

- Patients are taught to reconceptualise their pain by emphasising how it can be controlled by thoughts, feelings and beliefs.
- Imagery and diversion techniques are important.
- The practice and consolidation of these techniques in general situations are assessed.

KEY MESSAGE

The way a patient thinks about the pain will affect the extent and nature of their pain.

QUICK CHECK

What are cognitions and how do they contribute to pain?

THINK ABOUT THIS

How can we use cognitions and cognitive behavioural therapy to improve pain management? Talk to a person in pain and see what sort of thought processes the individual is going through.

Pain redefinition

The situation in a dentist's reception area outlined above is a good example of this technique. The patient is asked to redefine their pain in more positive terms, for example rather than something being painful they may find it easier to refer to it as unpleasant but necessary, or less unpleasant than . . . . Similarly, they may wish to redefine the sensation as a scratching or vibration, or hot/cold, rather than a feeling of pain.

Distraction

This is a technique where the focus of attention is away from the painful experience. For example, a nurse may encourage a child to look away from the needle while having an injection, or may distract them by asking them about a game or television programme they enjoy. This technique has been supported by recent research into the effects of television watching on reported pain by children during venipuncture (Bellieni *et al.*, 2006).

A strength of the distraction technique is that it is simple to administer, requiring no special training or equipment and can be used in multiple settings. As one may predict, this approach (like relaxation) can influence the success of a number of techniques and has been used to explain some and even all of the success of other pain reducing interventions, e.g. acupuncture.

QUICK CHECK

Where would you use the distraction technique and with what type of patient?

Imagery

Similar to this distraction technique is **imagery**. With this technique a patient is asked to focus on an imagined activity that makes them feel happy, pleasant or safe, as opposed to focusing on the situation around them. Images may include lying on a beach, walking through a meadow or sitting in their sister's living room on a noisy Christmas morning. The therapist may guide them through the process, asking them to pay attention to various sensations, smells, sounds, tastes; this can then be applied outside of the therapy session.

Group interventions

So far all of these techniques have been discussed on the basis of their application to individuals; however, a number of benefits have been identified in the administration of group therapy for those with chronic pain. The use of group interventions, particularly CBT group therapy, is becoming commonplace (Thorn and Kuhaida, 2006). It is suggested that these benefits may result from a number of factors:

● Putting an individual's pain up against others' helps them to realise the extent of their pain experience.

- Social support gained from this approach may improve opportunities for distractions and interest in other activities, thus reducing boredom and a focus on the pain experience alone.
- The group may provide positive reinforcement for reductions in negative pain behaviours such as avoidance and for an increase in positive behaviours such as returning to work or increased physical activity.

> **KEY MESSAGE**
> Using a range of methods to manage pain can be extremely beneficial.

7.10 Conclusion

Pain is one of the most common occurrences in healthcare and as such it is vital that nurses and all other healthcare professionals are aware of the factors influencing this experience. Previously the view of pain was merely as a medical perspective, but psychological factors are now recognised as having an important role to play in its experience. Consequently there are now numerous psychological approaches to the management of pain which can easily be incorporated, where necessary, into nursing care.

7.11 Summary

- The nature of pain is individual; varying in nature, pattern, severity and so on.
- There are many categories of pain representing some of these variations in the pain experience; chronic, acute, recurrent, progressive, intractable, benign.
- Early theories of pain proposed a direct link between injury and pain.
- Three groups of evidence bring early theories into question: (1) biological interventions successful at managing acute pain are sometimes ineffective with persistent pain; (2) the same injury in two individuals may produce different levels of pain; (3) phantom limb pain, pain without injury.
- Melzack and Wall proposed the gate control theory of pain which suggests there is a gate between injury and pain perception that moderates the level of perceived pain and is influenced by psychosocial as well as biological factors.
- Two frequently researched psychological factors of pain in current literature are coping styles and self-efficacy.

- There is no universally agreed objective measure of pain, but different measures for different patient groups with different forms of pain.

- Three dimensions of pain that most assessments consider are sensory, affective and impact.

- When designing an assessment this must be tailored to the individual.

- The most common form of assessment is verbal rating scales and these can be uni-dimensional (measuring one aspect of pain) or multidimensional (e.g. the McGill pain inventory).

- Interventions are designed to manage pain and are not considered a cure for this pain.

- The treatment of pain will vary depending on the type of pain presented.

- The most common intervention for pain is pharmacological. Although successful in the short term, there are associated problems such as tolerance and dependence.

- Behavioural interventions focus on reducing behaviours associated with pain and the involvement of family and friends is key to the success of this approach.

- Cognitive approaches to pain reduction focus on replacing or modifying thoughts around pain, e.g. through imagery, pain redefinition and distraction.

- Group interventions, particularly group CBT, are growing in popularity.

- Interventions are most often multi-modal in nature.

YOUR END POINT

Answer the following questions to assess your knowledge and understanding of pain and pain management.

1. Which of the following are tools used for pain assessment:

    (a) uni-dimensional

    (b) numerical

    (c) multidimensional

    (d) categorical

    (e) all of the above?

2. Which of the following pieces of evidence have been used to support the presence of psychological factors in the experience of pain:

    (a) people with amputated limbs can experience phantom limb pain

    (b) people can experience pain without injury

    (c) people differ in their perceptions of pain

    (d) people vary in the medication needed to relieve their pain

    (e) all of the above?

3. The linear-biomedical model of pain suggests that:

    (a) injury leads to pain signals

    (b) pain signals lead to the experience of pain

    (c) pain signals can be blocked

    (d) pain is an automatic response

    (e) all of the above.

4. Cognitive behavioural therapy can relieve pain through:

    (a) electrically stimulating muscle tissue around the source of the pain

    (b) changing the way a patient thinks about pain

    (c) slowly tensing and relaxing the muscles surrounding the painful area

    (d) negatively reinforcing pain behaviours

    (e) none of the above.

5. According to the gate controlled theory of pain, which factors open the pain gate:

    (a) depression

    (b) boredom

    (c) low activity levels

    (d) focusing on the pain

    (e) all of the above?

Further reading

Brodie, E., Whyte, A. and Niven, C. (2007). Analgesia through the looking-glass? A randomized controlled trial investigating the effect of viewing a 'virtual' limb upon phantom limb pain, sensation and movement. *European Journal of Pain*, 11(4), pp. 428–436.

Brodner, G., Mertes, N., Buerkle, H., Marcus, H.A.E. and Aken, H.V. (2000). Acute pain management: Analysis, implications and consequences after prospective experience with 6349 surgical patients. *European Journal of Anaesthesiology*, 17(9), pp. 566–575.

Melzack, R. and Wall, P. D. (1996). *The Challenge of Pain*. London: Penguin.

Morley, S., Eccleston, C. and Williams, A. (1999). Systematic review and meta-analysis of randomized controlled trials of cognitive behaviour therapy and behaviour therapy for chronic pain in adults, excluding headache. *Pain*, 80, pp. 1–13.

Morris, D.B. (1999). Sociocultural and religious meanings of pain. In R.J. Gatchel and D.C. Turk (eds), *Psychosocial Factors in Pain*. New York: Guilford Press.

Zhou, X. and Gao, D.G. (2008). Social support and money as pain management mechanisms. *Psychological Inquiry*, 19(3), pp. 127–144.

Weblinks

http://www.iasp-pain.org
International Association for the Study of Pain. This site provides detailed information on the study of pain and how this can be used to improve relief from pain.

http://pediatric-pain.ca
Paediatric pain. This site provides information on pain experienced by children. It includes links to paediatric pain research and self-help materials for families.

http://www.ampainsoc.org
American Pain Society. This site contains links to the latest pain research and news.

http://www.painsupport.co.uk/ps_home.html
Pain Support. This site provides detailed descriptions of a range of techniques that can be used to manage pain, including conventional medicine and alternative therapies.

http://www.biofeedbacktherapy.net
Biofeedback. This site contains detailed information on the biofeedback pain management technique.

Glossary

ABC model Model developed by Albert Ellis, characterised by a link between how an event is perceived and the behavioural and emotional consequences of that event.

Acupuncture The technique of using fine needles, positioned in specific areas of the body, as a means of stimulating the body's natural healing response in order to restore balance.

Acute pain A short-term pain arising from physical injury.

A-delta fibres Types of sensory fibres that relay pain information very quickly.

Anal stage Second stage of psychosexual development in which the ego is developed.

Behaviourism Movement in psychology, also known as the learning perspective: everything we do is the result of learning. A perspective aimed at transforming psychology into an objective science through the omission of subject matter that is not observable.

Biofeedback The technique of using feedback on activities within the body as a means of training individuals to control these activities.

Bottom-up processing Stimulus driven - directly affected by the stimulus you put in.

C fibres Slower sensory fibres.

Castration anxiety Phenomenon referred to in Freud's theory of psychosexual development, in which the son fears castration by his father as a result of his feelings towards his mother being uncovered.

Catharsis The release of emotional tension.

Central nervous system (CNS) A division of the nervous system made up of the brain and spinal cord.

Cerebral artery Arteries supply blood to the cerebral cortex.

Chunking Combining smaller pieces of information into larger chunks of information.

Classical conditioning etc. Associative learning in which a behaviour is learnt through its pairing with an unconditioned stimulus, eventually resulting in the learnt stimulus evoking a conditioned response in the absence of the unconditioned stimulus.

Cognitions Thought processes in which information is perceived, acknowledged and/or processed.

Cognitive dissonance Conflict or anxiety arising from the existence of two contradictory feelings, beliefs or actions.

Cognitive psychology Division of psychology focused on internal mental processing.

Cognitive revolution Stage in the history of psychology in which behaviourism (focused on objective observable phenomena) was replaced with an acceptance of the role of internal processes.

Cognitive behavioural therapy (CBT) Form of therapy that emphasises the role of thought in changing our behaviour and emotional responses.

Conditioned response A learnt response.

Conditioned stimulus A previously neutral stimulus which through associations with an unconditioned stimulus has become a trigger for a conditioned response.

Conscious A mental state in which events and thoughts are perceived.

Context-dependent learning Learning, the recall of which is dependent on the reproduction of certain aspects present in the context in which it was learnt.

Control methods A group that does not receive treatment in an experiment is known as the control group. This group receives a control method, a method similar to that of the treatment group but lacking the key component (e.g. a control method in an experiment looking at a new type of drug would be the distribution of a placebo to the control group).

Cortex The outer layer of the brain.

Cue A stimulus that provides information about what to do.

Defence mechanisms From Freudian theory, mental strategies for reducing the emotional distress experienced by the awareness of an unacceptable or traumatic thought or memory.

Demand characteristics Refers to the event in which a participant involved in experimental research interprets the purpose of the research and adjusts their response to the situation according to this interpretation.

Denial Rejection of information presented.

Deterministic Philosophical view that every event is caused by a preceding chain of events.

Displacement Emotions which cannot be directed at the person from which they stem are directed towards a substitute target.

Distraction Diversion of attention away from a given stimulus.

Dorsal horns One of the two roots of a spinal nerve that passes dorsally to the spinal cord and that consists of sensory fibres.

Echoic stores (auditory store) Store for auditory information.

Ecological validity Reflects real life situations and circumstances.

Ego One part of the personality as divided by Freud. Based on the reality principle, this component works to achieve the aims of the id in the long term, identifying and overcoming likely obstacles to this goal.

Electra complex Female equivalent of the Oedipus complex.

Electromyography (EMG) Measurement tool for assessing and recording activity levels in the muscles.

Emotion-focused coping Dealing with a problem by focusing on your emotional response to it.

Encoding The organisation of information into a form that can be retrieved and stored.

External LoC View that all actions are controlled by a force external to the individual such as luck.

Extinction Removal of a learnt response through a lack of reinforcement to the point that the association no longer exists.

Feminine Oedipus attitude Renamed as the Electra complex by Jung, this refers to the young girl's fixation on her father as a love interest.

Fixation Event in which the ego's energy is tied up with a conflict at a particular stage in psychosexual development resulting in the presentation of behaviours typical of this stage.

Gate control theory Theory of pain in which pain is the result of pain messages negotiated by a gate, which in turn is opened or closed by various biological, psychological and social factors.

Genital phase The final stage of psychosexual development as outlined by Freud.

Grey matter Mass of neuronal cell bodies.

Health belief model (HBM) A psychological model attempting to explain health behaviour through a consideration of perceived susceptibility, severity, benefits, barriers, cues and self-efficacy.

Health LoC The location in which control for health is placed, e.g. externally or internally.

Hypnosis The act of producing a suggested state similar to that of sleep.

Iconic store (visual store) Store for visual information.

Id The earliest component of personality, as identified in Freudian theory. Working on the pleasure principle, the id is responsible for attempting to fulfil instincts or natural drives through any means.

Idiographic approach Focuses on people as individuals with the view that no two people are alike.

Imagery The formation of mental images.

Information processing approach An approach within cognitive psychology which views the brain's function as that of a computer in order to understand human thinking.

Internal LoC View that all actions are controlled by the individual.

Introspection The study of human consciousness which involves research participants reporting on their own internal thought processes.

Latency period Fourth stage of psychosexual development, a rest period for the libido.

Law of effect View that responses which elicit a positive outcome will increase in frequency as a result of that positive outcome.

Learned helplessness Situation in which individuals or animals have learnt to act helpless in response to a given stimulus.

Linear-biomedical model One line or pathway which is biological in nature.

Locus of control (LoC) The location in which control for something is placed (e.g. externally or internally).

McGill pain questionnaire Multi-modal self-report pain survey.

Medical model Approach to an issue taken by Western medicine.

Memory The retention of and ability to recall information.

Modelling Responding to a given stimulus based on behaviours observed by another, also known as observational learning.

Multi-modal methods Use of a combination of more than one approach or model.

Negative reinforcement The absence or avoidance of a negative outcome or activity.

Nervous system Network of nerves.

Neurons Cells in the nervous system which relay information.

Neuropathic pain Pain occurring from within the nervous system itself which may originate from the peripheral nervous system or from the central nervous system.

Nociceptive pain Pain resulting from the stimulation of specific pain receptors.

Non-nociceptive Pain arising from within the **peripheral and central** nervous system.

Observational learning Learning through observing someone.

Oedipus complex Conflict within the phallic stage of psychosexual development in which the young boy fixates on his mother as a love interest.

Operants An influence, having an effect on something.

Oral stage First stage of psychosexual development, the outcome of which is predicted to influence trust factors in adult personality.

Paradigm A set of beliefs that are taken as fact, the generally accepted perspective in a discipline.

Penis envy Reaction by young girls to their realisation that they do not have a penis.

Phallic stage Third stage of psychosexual development in which the Oedipus and Electra complexes supposedly occur.

Phantom limbs Sensation emanating from an absent or removed limb suggesting the limb is still present.

Positive reinforcement Providing praise or reward for an action.

Pre-conscious Thoughts that are unconscious at a particular moment in time.

Primacy effect A tendency for the items near the beginning of the series to be better recalled than those near the middle.

Problem-focused approach Coping style which focuses on methods of solving the problem.

Progressive muscle relaxation (PMR) Technique in which individuals are relaxed by first tensing muscle groups and then paying attention to how the muscle relaxes.

Projection A defence mechanism in which one's own feelings and unwanted thoughts are projected onto someone else.

Psychic determinism A philosophical doctrine stating that all psychological and behavioural phenomena, such as human cognition, behaviour, decision, and action, are determined by the inevitable consequences of previous occurrences.

Psychoanalysis A system of ideas developed by Sigmund Freud, focusing on the development of abnormal personalities and developed through his work as a therapist.

Psychoanalytic theory Term referring to approaches to psychoanalysis based on empirical research.

Psychodynamic approach The theories and works of both Freud and his followers, all of whom view personality in relation to drives and instincts.

Psychopathology The study of mental illness or distress.

Rating scale A means of categorising pain via recording the person's perception of that pain on a scale.

Rational emotive (therapy) Framework founded by Ellis and applying the ABC model of thoughts and behaviours to therapy.

Reaction formation Defence mechanism in which unwanted thoughts or feelings are masked by extreme expressions of the opposite view.

Recency effect A tendency for the items near the end of the series to be better recalled than those near the start.

Reductionist The simplification of complex systems into interactions between smaller parts.

Reflexive response An instantaneous response sidetracking deep thought processes relating to how to respond.

Regression Refers to the movement backwards through the stages of psychosexual development.

Reinforcement An increase in the strength of a response as a result of the impact it has on the environment.

Reinforcement schedule When and how often a behaviour is reinforced. It can have a dramatic impact on the strength and rate of the response.

Reinforcer A stimulus that strengthens or weakens the behaviour that produced it.

Repression A form of defence mechanism in which unwanted or harmful information is removed from the conscious into the unconscious.

Retrieval The gathering of information.

Role schemas A collection of information relating to one's role within a given situation.

Schema A collection of information relating to a particular group of topics, an organisational structure for cognitions.

Script Information on the process of an action.

Self-efficacy The belief that one is capable of performing in a certain manner to attain certain goals.

Self-schemas Organisation of information relating to the self.

Serial processing Information units processed one after the other.

Social learning theory Theory focusing on the learning produced within a social context, seeing learning occurring through interactions and observations of others.

Somatic pain Detected with somatic nociceptors and present in ligaments.

Specificity theory Developed by Von Frey in 1894, assumes there are specific sensory receptors responsible for the transmission of sensation, warmth and pain.

Stereotyping Oversimplified descriptions of group members.

Stimulus generalisation The generalisation of a response to one stimulus to all stimuli that are similar to this conditioned stimulus.

Storage The holding of information.

Sublimation A defence in which unacceptable impulses are channelled through more acceptable behaviours.

Substantia gelatinosa Part of the posterior horn of the grey matter of the spinal cord.

Superego Final part of the personality to develop in Freud's personality theory, the superego refers to the conscience or inner parent that applies values and morality to the way in which we choose to act.

Sympathetic pain Pain that occurs due to possible over-activity of the sympathetic nervous system, and central/peripheral nervous system mechanisms.

Systematic desensitisation Type of behavioural therapy in which individuals are gradually presented with stimuli that more and more closely resemble their fear, in an attempt to reduce the anxiety provoked by this stimulus.

Tabula rasa view of mind View that the mind is a blank slate on which the experiences of life are written.

Talking cure Developed from treatment first piloted by Dr Breuer, refers to the process of talking that eventually reduced his patients' hysteria.

The protection motivation theory Proposes that health behaviours can be predicted on the basis of severity, susceptibility, response effectiveness and self-efficacy.

Top-down processing Concept driven and affected by what the individual contributes – information stored in the memory is used to interpret what is in front of you.

Transcranial doppler A test that measures the velocity of blood flow through the brain's blood vessels.

Transcutaneous electrical nerve stimulation (TENS) Application of electrical current through the skin for pain control.

Unconditioned response Innate response to a stimulus, such as fear or hunger.

Unconditioned stimulus Stimulus which naturally elicits a response such as food or a loud noise.

Unconscious Information to which we show no awareness.

Unstructured interview Interview with an individual, conducted without a requirement to stick to a plan of how content will be covered.

Verbal rating scale (VRS) A categorical assessment that involves patients rating their pain on a scale.

Vicarious reinforcement Reinforcement observed in another which will influence the observer's probability of completing the same reaction.

Visceral pain Pain occurring from stimulation of receptors within internal organs of the main body cavities. This pain originates from ongoing injury to the internal organs or the tissues that support them.

Visual analogue scale (VAS) A numerical assessment, involving patients rating their pain on a scale.

References

Action on Elder Abuse. (2004). *Hidden Voices*. London: Age Concern.

Adler, N. (2000). An international perspective on the barriers to the advancement of women managers. *Applied Psychology: An International Review*, 42, 289–300.

Adler, R. (1981). *Psychoneuroimmunology*. New York: Academic Press.

Adler, R., Felten, D.L. and Cohen, N. (eds) (2001). *Psychoneuroimmunology*, vol. 2. San Diego, CA: Academic Press.

Age Concern. (2006a). How Ageist is Britain? www.ageconcern.org.uk

Ajzen, I. (1985). From intentions to actions: A theory of planned behavior. In J. Kuhl and J. Beckmann (eds), *Action Control: From Cognition to Behavior*. Berlin, Heidelberg, New York: Springer-Verlag.

Ajzen, I. (1988). *Attitudes. Personality, and Behaviour*. Milton-Keynes, England: Open University Press.

Ajzen, I. and Fishbein, M. (1970). The prediction of behavior from attitudinal and normative variables. *Journal of Experimental Social Psychology*, 6, 466–487.

Alford, P. *et al.* (1995). Should nurses wear uniforms? *Nursing Standard*, 9, 52–53.

Andrasik, F. (2007). Efficacy of behavioural treatments for recurrent headaches. *Neurological Science*, 28, S70–S77.

Archer, J. (1999). *The Nature of Grief: The Evolution and Psychology of Reaction to Loss*. London: Routledge.

Argyle, M. (1988). *Bodily Communication*. London: Routledge.

Arkes, J.R., Boehm, L.E. and Xu, G. (1991). Determinants of judged validity. *Journal of Experimental Social Psychology*, 27, 576–605.

Arnett, J.J. (1999). Optimistic bias in adolescent and adult smokers and non smokers. *Addictive Behaviours*, 25(4), 625–632.

Asch, S.E. (1952). *Social Psychology*. Englewood Cliffs, NJ: Prentice Hall.

Atkinson, R.C. and Shiffrin, R.M. (1968). Human memory: A proposed system and its control processes. In K.W. Spence and J.T. Spence (eds), *The Psychology of Learning and Motivation*, vol. 8. London: Academic Press.

Ayman-Nolley S. and Taira L.L. (2000). Obsession with the dark side of adolescence: A decade of psychological studies. *Journal of Youth Studies*, 3, 35–48.

Bahrick, H.P., Bahrick, P.O. and Wittinger, R.P. (1975). Fifty years of memory for names and faces: A cross-sectional approach. *Journal of Experimental Psychology*, 104, 54–75.

Bandura, A. (1965). Influences of models' reinforcement contingencies on the acquisition of initiative responses. *Journal of Personality and Social Psychology*, 1, 589–593.

Bandura, A. (1977a). *Social Learning Theory*. Englewood Cliffs, NJ: Prentice Hall.

Bandura, A. (1977b). Self-efficacy: Toward a unifying theory of behavioural change. *Psychological Review*, 84(2), 191-215.

Bandura, A. (2000). Health promotion from the perspective of social cognitive theory. In P. Norman, C. Abraham and M. Connor (eds), *Understanding and Changing Health Behaviour: From Health Beliefs to Self-Regulation*, 229-242. Switzerland: Harwood Academic.

Bandura, A., Ross, D. and Ross, S.A. (1961). Transmission of aggression through imitation of aggressive models. *Journal of Abnormal and Social Psychology*, 63, pp. 575-582.

Barber, J. (1998). The mysterious persistence of hypnotic analgesia. *International Journal of Clinical and Experimental Hypnosis*, 46(1), 28-43.

Baron, R.A. (2001). *Psychology*, 5th edn. Boston, MA: Allyn and Bacon.

Becker, M. (1974). *The Health Belief Model and Personal Health Behavior*. Thorofare, NJ: Slack.

Beecher, H.K. (1959). Generalisation from pain of various types and diverse origins *Science*, 130, 267-268.

Bellieni, C.V., Cordelli, D.M., Raffaelli, M., Ricci, B., Morgese, G. and Buonocore, G. (2006). Analgesic effect of watching TV during venipuncture. *Archives of Disease in Childhood*, 91(12), 1015-1017.

Beltran, R.O., Scanlan, J.N., Hancock, N. and Luckett, T. (2007). The effect of first year mental health fieldwork on attitudes of occupational therapy students towards people with mental illness. *Australian Occupational Therapy Journal*, 54, 42-48.

Berkman, L.F. and Symes, S.L. (1979). Social networks, host-resistance, and mortality – 9 year follow up study of Alameda County residents. *American Journal of Epidemiology*, 109(2), 186-204.

Bibace, R. and Walsh, M.E. (1980). Development of children's concept of illness. *Paediatrics*, 66(6), 912-917.

Birch, S., Hesselink, J.K., Jonkman, F., Hekker, T. and Bos, A. (2004). Clinical research on acupuncture: Part 1. What have reviews of the efficacy and safety of acupuncture told us so far? *Journal of Alternative Complementary Medicine*, 10(3), 468-480.

Bovbjerg, D.H., Redd, W.H., Jacobsen, P.B., Manne, S.L., Taylor, K.L., Surbone, A. *et al.* (1992). An experimental analysis of classically conditioned nausea during cancer chemotherapy. *Psychosomatic Medicine*, 54(6), pp. 623-637.

Bowlby, J. (1969). *Attachment and Loss*. New York: Basic Books.

Bowling, A. (1995). *Measuring Disease*. Buckingham: Open University Press.

British Thoracic Society and Scottish Intercollegiate Guidelines Network (2003). *British Guideline on the Management of Asthma: A national clinical guideline*. Retrieved 24 May 2009, from http://www.brit-thoracic.org.uk/Portals/0/ Clinical%20Information/Asthma/Guidelines/asthma_final2008.pdf

Broadbent, D. (1958). *Perception and Communication*. London: Pergamon Press.

Brummett, B.H., Barefoot, J.C., Siegler, I.C., Clapp-Channing, N.E., Lytle, B.L.L., Bosworth, H.B., Williams, R.B. and Mark, D.B. (2001). Characteristics of socially isolated patients with coronary artery disease who are at elevated risk for mortality. *Psychosomatic Medicine*, 63(2), 267–272.

Bruner, J. (1983). Play, thought, and language. *Peabody Journal of Education*, 60(3), 60–69.

Bruster, S., Jarman, B., Bosanquet, N. *et al.* (1994). National survey for hospital patients. *British Medical Journal*, 309(6968), 1542–1546.

Bugental, J. (1965). *The Search for Authenticity: An Existential-Analytic Approach to Psychotherapy*. London: Holt, Rinehart and Winston.

Bunker, S.J., Colquhoun, D.M., Esler, M.D., Hickie, I.B., Hunt, D., Jelinek, V.M., Oldenburg, B.F., Peach, H.G., Ruth, D., Tennant, C.C. and Tonkin, A.M. (2003). Stress and coronary heart disease: Psychosocial risk factors. National Heart Foundation of Australia Position Statement Update. *Medical Journal of Australia*, 178(6), 272–276.

Burgess, L., Page, S. and Hardman, P. (2006). Changing attitudes in dementia care and the role of nurses. *Nursing Times*, 99(18).

Burish, T.G., Shartner, C.D. and Lyles, J.N. (1981). Effectiveness of multiple muscle-site EMG biofeedback and relaxation training in reducing the aversiveness of cancer chemotherapy. *Biofeedback and Self-Regulation*, 6(4), 523–535.

Bush, T. (2003). Communicating with patients who have dementia. *Nursing Times*, 99(42).

Cappell H. and Greeley J. (1987). Alcohol and tension reduction: An update on research and theory. In H.T. Blane and K.E. Leonard (eds), *Psychological Theories of Drinking and Alcoholism*, 15–54. New York: Guilford Press.

Carey, P. (1985). Manner and meaning in West Sumatra: The social-context of consciousness. *The Times Literary Supplement*, 4305, 112.

Caris-Verhallen, M., Kerkstra, A. and Bensing, J.M. (2001). Non-verbal behaviour in nurse-elderly patient communication. *Journal of Advanced Nursing*, 29(1), 808–818.

Carlson, N.R. and Buskist, W. (1997). *Psychology: The Science of Behaviour* (5th edn). Needham Heights, MA; Allyn and Bacon.

Cartwright, M., Wardle, J., Steggles, N., Simon, A.E., Croker, H. and Jarvis, M.J. (2003). Stress and Dietary Practices in Adolescents. *Health Psychology*, 22(4), 362–369.

Chen, C. and Farruggia, S. (2002). Culture and adolescent development. In W.J. Lonner, D.L. Dinnel, S.A. Hayes and D.N. Sattler (eds), *Online Readings in Psychology and Culture* (Unit 11, Chapter 2). Bellingham, Washington: Western Washington University, Center for Cross-Cultural Research. http://www.wwu.edu/~culture

Cherry, C. (1966). *On Human Communication: A Review , a Survey, and a Criticism*, 2nd edn. Cambridge, MA: MIT Press

Clark, A. (2003). 'It's like an explosion in your life...': Lay perspectives on stress and myocardial infraction. *Journal of Clinical Nursing*, 12, 544–553.

Cleland, J.A. Palmer, J.A. and Venzke, W.J. (2005). Ethnic differences in pain perception. *Physical Therapy Reviews*, 10, 113–122.

Cohen, L., Savary, C. and de Moor, C. (2000). Stress and social support affect immune function in cancer patients receiving vaccine treatment. *Psychosomatic Medicine*, 62(1), 1137.

Cohen, S. (2005). The Pittsburgh Common Cold Studies: Psychosocial predictors of susceptibility to respiratory infectious illness. *International Journal of Behavioural Medicine*, 12(3), 123–131.

Cohen, S., Frank, E., Doyle, W.J., Skoner, D.P., Rabin, B.S. and Gwaltney Jr, J.M. (1998). Types of stressors that increase susceptibility to the common cold In healthy adults. *Health Psychology*, 17(3), 214–223.

Cohn, N.J. and Squire, L.R. (1980). Preserved learning and retention of pattern-analyzing skill in amnesia: Dissociation of knowing how and knowing that. *Science*, 210(4466), 207–210.

Conner, M. and Norman, P. (1996). *Predicting Health Behavior. Search and Practice with Social Cognition Models*. Ballmore, Buckingham: Open University Press.

Coyne, I. (2006). Consultation with children in hospital: Children, patients' and nurses' perspectives. *Journal of Clinical Nursing*, 15, 61–71.

Craik, F.I.M. and Lockhart, R.S. (1972). Levels of processing: A framework for memory research. *Journal of Verbal Learning and Verbal Behavior*, 11, 671–684.

Cramer, J.A. and Rosenheck, R. (1998). Compliance with medication regimens for mental and physical disorders. *Psychiatry Service*, 49, 196–201.

Cumming, E. and Henry, W.E. (1961). *Growing Old: The Process of Disengagement*. New York: Basic Books.

Curran, J., Machin, C. and Gournay, K. (2006). Cognitive behavioural therapy for patients with anxiety and depression. *Nursing Standard*, 21(7), 44–52.

Dahlgren, G. and Whitehead, M. (1991). *Policies and strategies to promote social equity in health*. Stockholm: Institute of Futures Studies.

Dean, C. and Surtees, P.G. (1989). Do psychological factors predict survival in breast cancer? *Journal of Psychosomatic Research*, 33(5), 561–569.

Department of Health (DoH) (2001). *A Research and Development Strategy for Public Health*. London: Department of Health.

Department of Health (DoH) (2005a). *Creating a patient-led NHS: Delivering the NHS Improvement Plan*. London: Department of Health.

Department of Health (DoH) (2005b). *Independence, Well-being and Choice: Our Vision for the Future of Social Care for Adults in England*. London: Department of Health.

Department of Health (DoH) (2006). *Our health, our care, our say: a new direction for community services*. London: Department of Health.

Donovan, J.L. and Blake, D.R. (1992). Patient compliance: Deviance or reasoned decision making? *Social Science and Medicine*, 34, 507–513.

Durkin, K. (1995). *Developmental Social Psychology: From Infancy to Old Age*. Oxford: Wiley Blackwell.

Eiser, C. (1997). Children's quality of life measures. *Archives of Disease in Childhood*, 77, 350–354.

Eiser, C. (1989). Children's understanding of illness: A critique of the 'stage' approach. *Psychology and Health*, 3, 93–101.

Elfant, E., Burns, J.W. and Zeichner, A. (2008). Repressive coping style and suppression of pain-related thoughts: Effects on responses to acute pain induction. *Cognition and Emotion*, 22(4), 671–696.

Ellis, A. (1962). *Reason and Emotion in Psychotherapy*. Secaucus, NJ: Prentice-Hall.

Evans, D.L., Leserman, J., Perkins, D.O., Stern, R.A., Murphy C., Zheng, B., Gettes, D., Longmate, J.A., Silva, S.G., van der Horst, C.M., Hall, C.D., Folds, J.D., Golden, R.N. and Petitto, J.M. (1997). Severe life stress as a predictor of early disease Progression In HIV Infection. *American Journal of Psychiatry*, 154(5), 630–634.

Eyesenck, M.W. and Flanagan, C. (2007). *Psychology for A2 Level*. East Sussex: Psychology Press.

Feil, N. (1996). Validation: Techniques for communicating with confused old-old persons and improving their quality of life. *Topics in Geriatric Rehabilitation*, 11(4), 34–42.

Feldt, K.S. (2000). The Checklist of Nonverbal Pain Indicators (CNPI). *Pain Management Nursing*, 1(1), 13–21.

Ferns, T. (2007). Factors that influence aggressive behaviour in acute care settings. *Nursing Standard*, 21(33), pp. 41-45.

Festinger, L. (1957). *A Theory of Cognitive Dissonance*. Stanford CA: Stanford University Press.

Fishbein, M. (1967). Attitude and the prediction of behavior. In M. Fishbein (ed.), *Readings in Attitude Theory and Measurement*, 477–492. New York: Wiley.

Fishbein, M. and Ajzen, I. (1975). *Belief, Attitude, Intention, and Behavior: An Introduction to Theory and Research*. Ontario: Addison-Wesley.

Fiske, S.T. and Taylor, S.E. (1991). *Social Cognition* (2nd edn). New York: McGraw-Hill.

Folkman, S. and Lazarus, R.S. (1988). Coping as a mediator of emotion. *Journal of Personality and Social Psychology*, 54(3), 466–475.

Fordyce, W.E., Lansky, D., Calsyn, D.A., Shelton, J.l., Stolov, W.C. and Roch, D.I. (1984). Pain measurement and pain behaviour. *Pain*, 18(1), 53–69.

Frank, A.J.M., Moll, J.M.H. and Hort, J.F. (1982). A comparison of three ways of measuring pain. *Rheumatology*, 21, 211–217.

Frasure-Smith, N., Lesperance, F., Gravel, G., Masson, A., Juneau, M., Talajic, M. and Bourassa, M. G. (2000). Social support, depression, and mortality during the first year after myocardial infarction. *Circulation*, 101(16), 1919-1924.

French, S.E., Lenton, R., Walter, V. and Eyles, J. (2000). An empirical evaluation of an expanded nursing stress scale. *Journal of Nursing Measurement*, 8, 161–178.

Friedman, M. and Rosenman, R.H. (1974). *Type A behavior and your heart*. New York: Knopf.

Furlan, A.D., van Tulder, M., Cherkin, D., Tsukayama, H., Lao, L., Koes, B. and Berman, B. (2005). Acupuncture and dry-needling for low back pain: An updated systematic review within the framework of the Cochrane Collaboration. *Spine*, 30(8), 944-963.

Garrison, M.M., Christakis, D.A., Ebal, B.E. Wiehe, S.E. and Rivara, F.P. (2003). A systematic review of smoking cessation interventions for adolescents. *Paediatric Research*, 53(4), 3206.

Garsson, B. (2004). Psychological factors and cancer development: Evidence after 30 years of research. *Clinical Psychology Review*, 24(3), 315–338.

Gatchel, R.J., Bo Peng, Y., Peters, M.L., Fuchs, P.H. and Turk, D.C. (2007). The biopsychosocial approach to chronic pain: Scientific advances and future directions. *Psychological Bulletin*, 133, 581–624.

Gibson, P., Powell, H., Coughlan , J., Wilson, A.J., Abramson, M., Haywood, P., Bauman, A., Hensley, M.J. and Walters, E.H. (2002). Self-management education and regular practitioner review for adults with asthma. *Cochrane Database of Systematic Reviews*, Issue 3.

Glanzer, M. and Cunitz, A.R. (1966). Two storage mechanisms in free recall. *Journal of Verbal Learning and Verbal Behaviour*, 5, 351–360.

Goldschneider, A. (1920). *Das Schmerz Problem*. Berlin: Springer.

Goll, P.S. (2004). Mnemonic strategies: Creating schemata for learning enhancement. *Education*, 125(2), 306–314.

Graf, P. and Schacter, D.L. (1985). Implicit and explicit memory for new associations in normal and amnesic subjects. *Journal of Experimental Psychology: Learning, Memory, and Cognition*, 11, 501–518.

Gray-Toft, P. and Anderson, J.G. (1981). The Nursing Stress Scale: Development of an instrument. *Journal of Behavioural Assessment*, 3(1), 11–23.

Greenberger, E., Chen, C., Tally, S. and Dong, Q. (2000). Family, peer, and individual correlates of depressive symptomatology in U.S. and Chinese adolescents. *Journal of Consulting and Clinical Psychology*, 68, 202–219.

Greer, S., Morris, T., Pettingale, K.W. and Haybittle, J.L. (1990). Psychological responses to breast cancer: Effect on outcome. *Lancet*, 335(8680), 49–50.

Gregson, R.A.M. and Stacey, B.G. (1981). Components of some New Zealand attitudes to alcohol and drinking in 1978-79: A preliminary report. *New Zealand Psychologist*, 9, 29–33.

Gremigni, P., Bacchi, F., Turrini, C., Cappelli, G., Albertazzi, A., Enrico, P. and Bitti, R. (2007). Psychological factors associated with medication adherence following renal transplantation. *Clinical Transplantation*, 21(6), 710–715.

Gross, R. and Kinnison, N. (2007). *Psychology for Nurses and Allied Health Professionals*. London: Hodder Arnold.

Harlow, H.F. (1959). Love in infant monkeys. *Scientific American*, 200(6), 64–74.

Haynes, R.B., Taylor, D.W. and Sackett, D.L. (1979). *Compliance in healthcare*. Baltimore, MD: Johns Hopkins University Press.

Health and Age (2006). The importance of empathy when nursing patients. *Health and Age*, 27 November.

Heffer, K.L., Kiecolt-Glaser, J.K., Loving, T.J., Glaser, R. and Malarkey, W.B. (2004). Spousal support satisfaction as a modifier of physiological responses to marital conflict in younger and older couples. *Journal of Behavioural Medicine*, 27(3), 233–254.

Hellzen, O., Kristiansen, L. and Norbergh, K.G. (2003). Nurses' attitudes towards older residents with long-term schizophrenia. *Journal of Advanced Nursing Practice*, 43(6), 616–622.

Heslop, P., Smith, G.D., Carroll, D., Macleod, J., Hyland, F. and Hart, C. (2001). Perceived stress and coronary heart disease risk factors: The contribution of socio-economic position. *British Journal of Health Psychology*, 6(2), 167-178.

Hibbard, J.H. and Pope, C.R. (1993). The quality of social roles as predictors of morbidity and mortality. *Social Science and Medicine*, 36(3), 217-225.

Hogg, M.A. and Vaughan, G.M. (2005). *Social Psychology* (4th edn). Harlow: Pearson Education.

Holmes, T.H. and Rahe, R.H. (1967). The Social Readjustment Rating Scale. *Journal of Psychosomatic Research*, 11, 213-218.

Horne, R. and Weinmann, J. (1999). Patients' beliefs about prescribed medicines and their role in adherence to treatment in chronic physical illness. *Journal of Psychsomatic Research,* 47, 555-567.

Hough, M. (2002). *A Practical Approach to Counselling.* Harlow: Pearson Education.

Houldin, A.D. (2000). *Patients with cancer: Understanding psychological pain.* Philadelphia: Lippincott Williams and Wilkins.

Houts, P.S., Doak, C.C., Doak, L.G. and Loscalzoc, M.G. (2006). The role of pictures in improving health communication: A review of research on attention, comprehension, recall, and adherence, *Patient Education and Counseling*, 61(2), 173-190.

Hovland, C.I., Janis, I.L. and Kelley, H.H. (1953). *Communication and Persuasion.* New Haven, CT: Yale University Press.

HSE. (2005). Psychosocial Working Conditions in Great Britain in 2005. Health and Safety Executive. Retrieved 18 November 2008, from http://www.hse.gov.uk/statistics/causdis/pwc2005.pdf

Hunt, P. and Pearson, D. (2001). Motivating change. *Nursing Standard*, 16(2), 45-52.

Huque, M.F. (1988). Experiences with meta-analysis in NDA submissions. *Proceedings of the Biopharmaceutical Section of the American Statistical Association*, 2, 28-33.

IASP. (1992). *Classification of Chronic Pain* (2nd edn). Seattle: International Association for the Study of Pain, IASP.

Iliffe, S. and Drennan, V. (2001). *Primary Care and Dementia*. London: Jessica Kingsley.

Jacobson, E. (1938). *Progressive Relaxation*. Chicago: University of Chicago Press.

Janis, I.L. (1967). Effect of fear arousal on attitude change: Recent developments in theory and experimental research. In L. Berkowitz (ed.), *Advances in Experimental Social Psychology*, 167-224. New York: Academic Press.

Jones, H. (1993). Altered images. *Nursing Times*, 89(5), 58-60.

Jones, J.R., Huxtable, C.S. and Hodgson, J.T. (2006). *Self-Reported Work-Related Illness in 2004/05: Results from The Labour Force Survey.* Caerphilly: Health and Safety Executive.

Jones, S.E. and Yarbrough, A.E. (1985). A naturalistic study of the meanings of touch. *Communication Monographs*, 52, 19-56.

Karling, M., Renstrom, M. and Ljungman, G. (2002). Acute and postoperative Pain in children. *Acta Paediatric*, 91(6), 660-666.

Kastenbaum, R. (1979). *Growing Old - Years of Fulfilment*. London: Harper and Row.

Kater, K.J., Rohwer, J. and Levine, M.P. (2000). An elementary school project for developing healthy body image and reducing the risk factors for unhealthy and disordered eating. *Eating Disorders*, 3-15.

Keller, P.A. and Block, L.G. (1995). Increasing the persuasiveness of fear appeals: The effect of arousal and elaboration. *Journal of Consumer Research*, 22, 448-459.

Kelly, J. (1995). Making sense of drug compliance. *Nursing Times*, 91(40), 40-41.

Kemeny, M.E. (2003). The psychology of stress. *Current Directions in Psychological Science*, 12(4), 124-129.

Kessels, R.P.C. (2003). Patients' memory for medical information. *Journal of Royal Society Medicine*, 96, 219-222.

Khadilkar, A., Odebiyi, D.O., Brosseau, L. and Wells, G.A. (2008). Transcutaneous Electrical Nerve Stimulation (TENS) versus placebo for chronic low-back pain. *Physical Therapy Reviews*, 13(5), 355-365.

Kiecolt-Glaser, J.K., Fisher, L.D., Ogrocki, P., Stout, J.C., Speicher, C.E. and Glaser, R. (1987). Marital quality, marital disruption, and immune function. *Psychosomatic Medicine*, 49(1), 13-34.

Kiecolt-Glaser, J.K. and Glaser, R. (1992). Psychoneuroimmunology: Can psychological interventions modulate immunity? *Journal of Consulting and Clinical Psychology*, 60(4), 569-575.

Kiecolt-Glaser, J.K., Loving, T.J., Stowell, J.R., Malarkey, W.B., Lemeshow, S., Dickinson, S.L. and Glaser, R. (2005). Hostile marital interactions, proflammatory cyrokine production, and wound healing. *Archives of General Psychiatry*, 62, 1377-1384.

King-Sears, M.E., Mercer, C.D. and Sindelar, P.T. (1992). Toward independence with keyword mnemonics: A strategy for science vocabulary instruction. *Remedial and Special Education*, 13(5), 22-33.

Kitwood, T. (1997). *Dementia Reconsidered: The Person Comes First*. Buckingham: Open University Press.

Kobasa, S.C. (1979). Stressful life events, personality, and health: Inquiry into hardiness. *Journal of Personality and Social Psychology*, 37(1), 1-11.

Kreitler, S. (1999). Denial in cancer patients. *Cancer Investigation*, 17, 514-534.

Kreuter, M.W., Chheda, S.G. and Bull, F.C. (2000). How does physician advice influence patient behaviour? *Archives of Family Medicine*, 9, 426-433.

Kübler-Ross, E. (1969). *On Death and Dying*. New York: Macmillan.

Kuhn, S., Cooke, K., Collins, M., Jones, J.M. and Mucklow, J.C. (1990). Perceptions of pain after surgery. *British Medical Journal*, 300, 1687-1690.

Lam, D. and Gale, J. (2000). Cognitive behaviour therapy: Teaching a client the ABC model - the first steps towards the process of change. *Journal of Advanced Nursing*, 31(2), 444-451.

Langley, P., Fonseca, J. and Iphofen, R. (2006). Psychoimmunology and health from a nursing perspective. *British Journal of Nursing*, 15(20), 1126-1129.

Launder, W., Davidson, G., Anderson, I. and Barclay, A. (2005). Self-neglect: The role of judgments and applied ethics. *Nursing Standard*, 19(18), 45-51.

Lavoie. A. (2008). Pain hurts more if the person hurting you means it. Retrieved 20 January 2009, from http://www.medicalnewstoday.com/articles/133127.php

Lazarus, R.S. and Folkman, S. (1984). *Stress, Appraisal, and Coping*. New York: Springer.

Lazarus, R.S. and Folkman, S. (1987). Transactional theory and research on emotions and coping. *European Journal of Personality*, 1, 141–170.

Lee, M. and Rotheram-Borus, M.J. (2001). Challenges associated with increased survival among parents living with HIV. *American Journal of Public Health*, 91(8), 1303–1309.

Lerner, R.M., Villarruel, F.A. and Castellino, D.R. (1999). *Adolescence: Developmental Issues in the Clinical Treatment of Children*, 125–136. Boston, MA: Allyn and Bacon.

Leserman, J. (2003). HIV disease progression: Depression, stress and possible mechanisms. *Biological Psychiatry*, 54(3), 295–306.

Levy-Storms, L. (2008). Therapeutic communication training in long-term care institutions: Recommendations for future research. *Patient Education and Counseling*, 73(1), 8–21.

Lewin, K. (1946). Action research and minority problems. In E. Hart and M. Bond (eds), *Action Research for Health and Social Care: A Guide to Practice*. Buckingham: Open University Press.

Ley, P. (1979). Memory for medical information. *British Journal of Social Clinical Psychology*, 18, 245–255.

Ley, P. (1981). Professional non-compliance: A neglected problem. *British Journal of Clinical Psychology*, 20, 151–154.

Ley, P. (1989). Improving patients' understanding, recall, satisfaction and compliance. In A. Boome (ed.), *Health Psychology*. London: Chapman and Hall.

Liddell, C., Rae, G., Brown, T.R, Johnston, D., Coates, V. and Mallet, J. (2004). Giving patients an audiotape of their GP consultation: A randomized control trial. *British Journal of General Practice*, 54(506), 667–672.

Lillberg, K., Verkasalo, P.K., Kapiro, J., Teppo, L., Helenius, H. and Koskenvuo, M. (2003). Stressful life events and risk of breast cancer in 10,808 women: A cohort study. *American Journal of Epidemiology*, 157, 415–423.

Lin, M.F., Chiou, J.H., Chou, M.H. and Hsu, M.C. (2006). Significant experience of token therapy from the perspective of psychotic patients. *Journal of Nursing Research*, 14(4), 315–323.

Lingam, R. and Scott, J. (2003). Treatment non-adherence in affective disorders. *Acta Psychiatrica Scandinavica*, 105(3), 164–172

Lowe, G. (1995). Alcohol and drug addiction. In A.A. Lazarus and A.M. Coleman (eds), *Abnormal Psychology*. London: Longman.

Lumsdaine, A.A. and Janis, I. L. (1953). Resistance to 'counterproperganda' produced by one-sided and two-sided 'propoganda' presentations. *Public Opinion Quarterly*, 17, 311–318.

Lundberg, U. (2006). Stress subjective and objective health. *International Journal of Social Welfare*, 15(1) (suppl.), s41–s48.

Marks, D.F. (2005). *Health Psychology: Theory, Research and Practice*. London: Sage.

Maslow, A. (1954). *Motivation and personality*. New York: Harper and Row.

Masse, R. (2000). Qualitative and quantitative analyses of psychological distress: methodological complementarity and ontological incommensureability. *Qualitative Health Research*, 10(3), 411-423

Matarazzo, J.D. (1982). Behavioural health's challenge to academic, scientific and professional psychology. *American Psychologist*, 37, 1-14.

McAllister-Williams, R.H., Foran, K., Forrest, S., Ingram, G., McMahon, L., Taylor, M., Rajwal, M. and Cornwall, L. (2006). NICE guidelines on antidepressants. *British Journal of General Practice*, 56(531),798-800.

McDonald, H.P., Garg, A.X. and Haynes, R.B. (2002). Interventions to enhance patient adherence to medication prescriptions: Scientific review. *Journal of the American Medical Association*, 288, 2868-2879.

McGregor, B.A., Antoni, M.H., Boyers, A., Alferi, S.M., Blomberg, B.B. and Carver, C.S. (2004). Cognitive-behavioural stress management increases benefit finding and immune function among women with early-stage cancer. *Journal of Psychosomatic Research*, 56(1), 1-8.

McGuire, W.J. (1969). The nature of attitude and attitude change. In G. Lindzey and E. Aronson (eds, 2nd edn), *Handbook of Social Psychology*, vol. 3. Reading, MA: Addison-Wesley.

McGuire, W.J. (1986). The vicissitudes of attitudes and similar representational constructs in twentieth century psychology. *European Journal of Social Psychology*, 16, 89-130.

Mearns, J. (2008). *The Social Learning Theory of Julian B. Rotter*. Retrieved 12 January 2009 from http://psych.fullerton.edu/jmearns/rotter.htm

Meichenbaum, D.M. and Cameron, R. (1983). Stress inoculation training: Toward a general paradigm for training coping skills. In D. Meichenbaum and M.E. Jaremko (eds), *Stress Reduction and Prevention*. New York: Plenum.

Melamed, B.G., Hawes, R.R., Heiby, E. and Gluck, J. (1975). Use of filmed modelling to reduce uncooperative behaviour of children during dental treatment. *Journal of Dental Research*, 54(4), 797-801.

Melzack, R. (1975). The McGill Pain Questionnaire: Major properties and scoring methods. *Pain*, 1, 277-299.

Melzack, R. and Wall, P.D. (1965). Pain mechanisms: A new theory. *Science*, 150, 971-979.

Melzack, R. and Wall, P.D. (1973). *The Challenge of Pain*. New York: Basic Books.

Metcalf, C., Smith, G.D., Wadsworth, E. *et al.* (2003). A contemporary validation of the Reeder Stress Inventory. *British Journal of Health Psychology*, 8, 83-94.

Milgram. S (1963). Behavioural Study of Obedience. *Journal of Abnormal and Social Psychology*, 67, 371-378.

Miller, E. and Morris, R. (1993). *The Psychology of Dementia*. Chichester: Wiley.

Miller, G.A. (1956). The magical number seven, plus or minus two: Some limits on our capacity for processing information. *Psychological Review*, 63, 81-97.

Miller, W.R. and Rollnick, S. (2002). *Motivational Interviewing: Preparing People for Change*. New York: Guildford Press.

Montgomery, G.H. and Bovbjerg, D.H. (1997). The development of anticipatory nausea in patients receiving adjuvant chemotherapy for breast cancer. *Physiology and Behaviour*, 61(5), 737–741.

Morrow, G.R. and Dobkin, P.L. (1988). Anticipatory nausea and vomiting in cancer patients undergoing chemotherapy treatment; prevalence, aetiology and behavioural interventions. *Clinical Psychology Review*, 8, 517–556.

Morrow, G.R. and Morrell, C. (1982). Behavioural treatment for the anticipatory nausea and vomiting induced by cancer chemotherapy. *New England Journal of Medicine*, 307(24), 1476–1480.

Morrow, G.R. and Rosenthal, S.N. (1996). Models, mechanisms and management of anticipatory nausea and emesis. *Oncology*, 53(Suppl 1), 4–7.

Morrow, G.R., Roscoe, J.A., Kirshner, J.J., Hynes, H.E. and Rosenbluth, R.J. (1998). Anticipatory nausea and vomiting in the era of 5-HT3 antiemetics. *Support Care Cancer,* 6(3), 244–247.

Morton, I. (1997). Beyond validation. In I.N. Norman and S.J. Redfern (eds), *Mental Health Care for Elderly People*. Edinburgh: Churchill Livingstone.

Morton I. (1999). *Person-Centred Approaches to Dementia Care*. Bicester: Winslow.

Murray, C.J. and Main, A. (2005). Role modelling as a teaching method for student mentors. *Nursing Times*, 101(26), 30–33.

Myant, K.A. and Williams, J.M. (2005). Children's concept of health and illness: Understanding of contagious illnesses, non-contagious illnesses and injuries. *Journal of Health Psychology*, 10(6), 805–819.

Neisser, U. (1967). *Cognitive Psychology*. Englewood Cliffs, NJ: Prentice-Hall.

Nishizawa, Y., Saito, M., Ogura, N., Kudo, S., Saito, K. and Hanaya, M. (2006). The non-verbal communication skills of nursing students: Analysis of interpersonal behavior using videotaped recordings in a 5-minute interaction with a simulated patient. *Japan Journal of Nursing Science*, 3, 15–22.

Norman, P. and Bennett, P. (1995). Health locus of control. In M. Conner and P. Norman (eds), *Predicting Health Behaviour,* 62–94. Buckingham: Open University Press.

Nursing and Midwifery Council (2008). *The Code: Standards of Conduct, Performance and Ethics for Nurses and Midwives. Standards 04.08*.

Odell, J. and Holbrook, J. (2006). Improving the hospital experience for older people. *Nursing Times*, 102(23), 23–24.

Ogden, J. (2004). *Health Psychology: A Textbook* (3rd edn). Oxford: Open University Press.

Ogden, J. (2007). *Health Psychology: A Textbook* (4th edn). England: Open University Press.

Oldham, A. (2007). Changing behaviour: Cognitive behavioural therapy: Linking thoughts and actions. *Journal of Primary Care Nursing*, 4(1), 26–29.

Oliver, S. and Ryan, S. (2004). Effective pain management for patients with arthritis. *Nursing Standard*, 18(50), 43–52.

Olsen, J. (1997). Nurse expressed empathy, patient outcomes and development of a middle range theory. *Journal of Nursing Scholarship*, 29(1), 71-76.

Ost, L.G. and Hugdahl, K. (1985). Acquisition of blood and dental phobia and anxiety response patterns in clinical patients. *Behaviour Research and Therapy*, 23(1), 27-34.

Palviainen, P., Hietala, M., Routasalo, P., Suominen, T. and Hupli, M. (2003). Do nurses exercise power in basic care situations? *Nursing Ethics*, 10(3).

Park, D.C., Morrell, R.W., Frieske, D. and Kincaid, D. (1992). Medication adherence behaviors in older adults: Effects of external cognitive supports. *Psychology and Aging*, 7, 252-256.

Parkes, C.M. (1972). *Bereavement, Studies of Grief in Adult Life*. Harmondsworth: Penguin.

Parkes, C.M. (1986). *Bereavement, Studies of Grief in Adult Life*. London: Tavistock.

Patterson, D.R., Wiechman, S.A., Jensen, M. and Sharar, S.R. (2006). Hypnosis delivered through virtual reality for burn pain: A clinical case series. *International Journal of Clinical and Experimental Hypnosis*, 54, 130-42.

Paul, G.L. and Lentz, R.J. (1977). *Psychosocial Treatment of Chronic Mental Patients: Milieu versus Social Learning Programs*. Cambridge, MA: Harvard University Press.

Pearcey, P.A. and Elliot, B.E. (2004). Student impressions of clinical nursing. *Nurse Education Today*, 24(5), 382-387.

Piaget, J. (1972). Intellectual evolution from adolescence to adulthood. *Human Development*, 15(1), 1-8.

Piaget, J. and Inhelder, B. (1956). *The Child's Conception of Space*. London: Routledge.

Population Trends. (2000). (PP2) 98/1. Official National Statistics, Annual Abstract for Statistics. Economics of Health Care. The Aging Population. Retrieved 5 September 2006, from http://www.oheschools.org/ohech6pg3.html

Price, B. (2006). Exploring person-centred care. *Nursing Standards*, 20(50), 49-56.

Prochaska J.O. and DiClemente C.C. (1982). Transtheoretical therapy: Toward a more integrative model of change. *Psychotherapy: Theory, Research and Practice*, 19, 276-288.

Rahman, A., Reed, E., Underwood, M., Shipley, M.E. and Omar, R.Z. (2008). Factors affecting self-efficacy and pain intensity In patients with chronic musculoskeletal pain seen in a specialist rheumatology pain clinic. *Rheumatology*, 47(12), 1803-1803.

Rains, J.C., Penzien, D.B. and Lipchik, G.L. (2006). Behavoral facilitation of medical treatment of headache: Implications of non-compliance and strategies for improving adherence. *Headache*, 46(5), 5142-5143.

Rana, D. and Upton, D. (2009). *Psychology for Nurses*. Harlow, UK: Pearson Education.

Raudonis, B.M. and Acton, G.J. (1997). Theory-based nursing practice. *Journal of Advanced Nursing*, 26(1), 138-145.

Raven, B.H. (1965). Social influence and power. In I.D. Steiner and M. Fishbein (eds), *Current Studies in Social Psychology*, 371-382. New York: Holt, Rinehart and Winston.

Reynolds, M. (2002). Reflecting on paediatric oncology nursing practice using Benner's helping role as a framework to examine aspects of caring. *European Journal of Oncology Nursing,* 6(1), 30–36.

Roelofs, J., Peters, M.L., De Jong, J.R. and Vlaeyen, J.W.S. (2002). Psychological treatment for chronic low back pain: Past, present and beyond. *Pain Reviews,* 9(1), 29–40.

Rogers, C. (1959). A theory of therapy, personality and interpersonal relationships as developed in the client-centered framework. In S. Koch (ed.). *Psychology: A Study of a Science. Vol. 3: Formulations of the Person and the Social Context.* New York: McGraw Hill.

Rogers, R.W. (1975). A protection motivation theory of fear appeals and attitude change. *Journal of Psychology,* 91, 93–114.

Rogers, R.W. (1983). Cognitive and physiological processes in fear appeals and attitude change: A revised theory of protection motivation. In J. Cacioppo and R. Petty (eds), *Social Psychophysiology.* New York: Guilford Press.

Roper, N. *et al.* (eds). (1983). *Using a Model for Nursing.* Edinburgh: Churchill Livingstone.

Rosenman, R.H., Friedman, M., Straus, R., Wurm, M., Kositchek, R., Haan, W. and Werthessen, N.T. (1964). A predictive study of coronary heart disease: The Western Collaborative Group Study. *Journal of the American Medical Association,* 189, 15.

Rosenstock, I. (1974). Historical origins of the Health Belief Model. *Health Education Monographs,* 2(4), 10.

Rosenthal, R. and Jacobson, L. (1968). *Pygmalion in the Classroom: Teachers' Expectations and Pupils' Intellectual Development.* New York: Holt.

Rothman, A.J. and Salovey, P. (1997). Shaping perception to motivate healthy behaviour: The role of message framing. *Psychological Bulletin,* 121, 3–19.

Rotter, J.B. (1954). *Social Learning and Clinical Psychology.* New York: Prentice Hall.

Rotter, J.B. (1966). Generalized expectancies for internal versus external control of reinforcement. *Psychological Monographs,* 80(609).

Royal College of Physicians, British Geriatrics Society, British Pain Society. (2007). *The Assessment of Pain in Older People; National Guidelines.* Concise guidance on good practice series, 8. London: RCP.

Russell, S., Daly, J., Hughes, E. and Hogg, C.O. (2003). Nurses and 'difficult' patients: Negotiating non-compliance. *Journal of Advanced Nursing,* 43(3), 281–287.

Ryle, G. (1949). *The Concept of Mind.* London: Hutchinson.

Sarafino, E.P. and Goehring, P. (2000). Age comparisons in acquiring biofeedback control and success in reducing headache pain. *Annals of Behavioural Medicine,* 22(1), 127–139.

Sarason, I.G., Levine, H.M., Basham, R.B. and Sarason, B.R. (1983). Assessing social support – The Social Support Questionnaire. *Journal of Personality and Social Psychology,* 44(1), 127–139.

Schaie K.W. and Willis, S.L. (2002). *Adult Development and Aging.* New York: Prentice Hall.

Schapiro, I.R., Ross-Petersen, L., Saelan, H., Garde, K., Olsen, J.H. and Johnsen, C. (2001). Extroversion and neuroticism and the associated risk of cancer: A danish cohort study. *American Journal of Epidemiology*, 153(8), 757-763.

Schneiderman, N., Ironson, G. and Siegel, S, D. (2005). Stress and health: Psychological, behavioural and biological determinants. *Annual Review of Clinical Psychology*, 1, 607-628.

Scott, J., Harmsen, M., Prictor, M.J., Entwistle, V.A., Snowden, A.J. and Watt, I. (2006). Recordings or summaries of consultations for people with cancer (Cochrane Review). *The Cochrane Library*, Issue 3. Oxford: Update Software/ Chichester: John Wiley.

Selye, H. (1956). What is stress? *Metabolism*, 5(5), 525-530.

Siegrist, J. and Marmot, M. (2004). Health inequalities and the psychosocial environment – two scientific challenges. *Social Science and Medicine*, 58(8) 1463-1473.

SIGN (2007). *Risk Estimation and the Prevention of Cardiovascular Disease. A National Clinical Guideline*. Retrieved 18 November 2008, from http://www.sign.ac.uk/pdf/sign97.pdf

Slater, R. (1995). *The Psychology of Growing Old: Looking Forward. Rethinking Ageing*. Buckingham: Open University Press.

Snelgrove, S. (2006). Factors contributing to poor concordance in health care. *Nursing Times*, 102(2).

Snowden, A. (2008). Medication management in older adults: A critique of concordance. *British Journal of Nursing*, 17(2), 114-121.

Spanos, N.P. and Katsanis, J. (1989). Effects of instructional set on attributions of nonvolition during hypnotic and nonhypnotic analgesia. *Journal of Personality and Social Psychology*, 56(2), 182-188.

Stockhorst, U., Klosterhalfen, S. and Steingruber, H.J. (1998). Conditioned nausea and further side-effects in cancer chemotherapy: A review. *Journal of Psychophysiology*, 12(suppl 1), 14-33.

Stroebe, M.S. (1998). New directions in bereavement research: Exploration of gender differences. *Palliative Medicine*, 12, 5-12.

Stroebe, W. (2000). *Social Psychology and Health* (2nd edn). Buckingham, UK: Open University Press.

Stuart-Hamilton, I. (1997). Adjusting to later life. *Psychology Review*, 4(2), 20-23.

Stuart-Hamilton, I. (2007). *Dictionary of Psychological Testing, Assessment and Treatment*. London: Jessica Kingsley Publishers.

Takano, Y. and Sogon, S. (2008). Are Japanese more collectivistic than Americans? Examining conformity in in-groups and the reference-group effect. *Journal of Cross-Cultural Psychology*, 39(3), 237-250.

Thomas, R., Daly, M., Perryman, B. and Stockton, D. (2000). Forewarned is forearmed – benefits of preparatory information on video cassette for patients receiving chemotherapy or radiotherapy – a randomised controlled trial. *European Journal of Cancer*, 356, 1536-1543.

Thorn, B.E. and Kuhajda, M.C. (2006). Group cognitive therapy for chronic pain. *Journal of Clinical Psychology: In Session*, 62(11), 1355-1366.

Townsend, E., Dimigen, G. and Fung D. (2000). A clinical study of child dental anxiety. *Behaviour Research and Therapy*, 38(1), 31-46.

Tulving, E. (1972). Episodic and semantic memory. In E. Tulving and W. Donaldson (eds), *Organization of memory*, 381-403. New York: Academic Press.

Uchino, B.N. (2004). *Social Support and Physical Health: Understanding the Health Consequences of Relationships*. New Haven, CT: Yale University Press.

Vasudeva, S., Claggett, A.L., Tietjen, G.E. and McGrady, A.V. (2003). Biofeedback – assisted relaxation in migraine headache: Relationship to cerebral blood flow velocity in the middle cerebral artery. *Headache: The Journal of Head and Face*, 43(3), 245-250.

Vygotsky, L.S. (1978). *Mind and Society: The Development of Higher Psychological Processes*. Cambridge, MA: Harvard University Press.

Wade, C. and Tavris, C. (2003). *Psychology* (7th edn). Upper Saddle River, NJ: Pearson Education Inc., Prentice Hall.

Waitzkin, H. (1989). A critical theory of medicine discourse. *Journal of Health and Social Behaviour*, 30, 220-239.

Wallston, K.A. and Wallston, B.S. (1982). Who is responsible for your health: The construct of health locus of control. In G. Sanders and J. Suls (eds), *Social Psychology of Health and Illness*, 65-98. Hillsadle, NJ: Lawrence Erlbaum and Associates.

Watson, J.B. (1913). Psychology as the behaviorist views it. *Psychological Review*, 20, 158-177.

Weiss, G.L. and Larsen, D.L. (1990). Health value, health locus of control and the prediction of health protective behaviours. *Social Behaviour and Personality*, 18(1), 121-136.

Weiss, M. and Britten, N. (2003). What is concordance? *The Pharmaceutical Journal*, 271(7270), 493.

Whitcher, S.J. and Fisher, J.D. (1979). Multidimensional reaction to therapeutic touch in a hospital setting. *Journal of Personality and Social Psychology*, 37, 87-96.

Wieland, D. (2000). Abuse of older persons: An overview. *Holistic Nursing Practice*, 14(4), 40-50.

Wilkin, H. and Silvester, J. (2007). *Nurses lacking empathy lower patient confidence*. Paper presented at the British Psychological Society's division of Occupational Psychology Annual Conference, Bristol.

Wolf, M.H., Putnam, S.M., James, S.A. and Stiles, W.B. (1978). The Medical Interview Satisfaction Scale: Development of a scale to measure patient perceptions physician behaviour. *Journal of Behaviour Medicine*, 1, 391-401.

Wong, D.L., Hockenberry-Eaton, M., Wilson, D., Winkelstein M.L. and Schwartz, P. (2001). *Wong's Essentials Of Pediatric Nursing* (6th edn). St Louis: Mosby Inc.

Workman, E.A. and La Via, M.F. (1987). T-Lymphocyte polyclonal proliferation: Effects of stress and stress response style on medical students taking National Board examinations. *Clinical Immunology and Immunopathology*, 43(3), 308-313.

World Health Organisation. (1946). Preamble to the Constitution of the World Health Organization as adopted by the International Health Conference, New York, 19-22 June. *Official Records of the World Health Organization*, 2, pp. 100.

World Health Organisation. (1993). The ICD-10. *The Classification of Mental and Behavioural Disorders*. Geneva: World Health Organisation.

Yehuda, R. and McEwen, B. (2004). Biobehavioral stress response - protective and damaging effects - introduction. *Annals of the New York Academy of Sciences*, 1032, XI-XVI.

Index